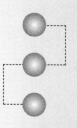

Endocrinology Science and Medicine

A Review of
Fundamental Principles

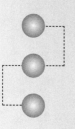

Endocrinology Science and Medicine

A Review of
Fundamental Principles

E. Victor Adlin, M.D.
Associate Professor Emeritus
Section of Endocrinology and Metabolism
Department of Medicine
Temple University School of Medicine

Series Editor

Michael A. Grippi, M.D.
Vice Chairman, Department of Medicine
Associate Professor of Medicine
Pulmonary, Allergy and Critical Care Division
University of Pennsylvania School of Medicine

Chief of Medicine
Veterans Administration Medical Center
Philadelphia, Pennsylvania

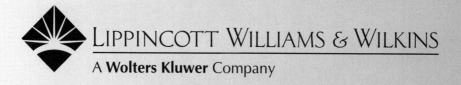

LIPPINCOTT WILLIAMS & WILKINS
A **Wolters Kluwer** Company

Editor: Elizabeth A. Nieginski
Editorial Director: Julie P. Scardiglia
Marketing Manager: Kelley Ray
Editorial Production: Shepherd, Inc.
Production Editor: Doug Nalean-Carlson

To purchase additional copies of this book call our customer service department at **(800) 638-3030** or fax orders to **(301) 824-7390**. International customers should call **(301) 714-2324**.

01 02
1 2 3 4 5 6 7 8 9 10

...... To Arlie, to Mike, and to Bill

Preface

Understanding clinical disorders requires a knowledge of the basic sciences; in no field of medicine is this truer than in endocrinology. This book aims to provide a brief review of the anatomy, biochemistry, and physiology of the major endocrine systems; to show how disturbances in the production and action of hormones can cause disease; and to relate these concepts to the diagnosis and management of the more common endocrine disorders.

Writing a small book on a big topic is difficult because of the many decisions that must be made to leave out potentially useful information. In making these decisions I have been guided mainly by the book's subtitle, "A Review of Fundamental Principles." But I have also considered whether a problem is commonly encountered in practice, and whether special difficulties exist in the understanding of a concept. For example, I have devoted more space than might seem necessary to describing the T_3-uptake test because physicians encounter this test in daily practice when they order certain "thyroid panels," and because students and physicians often (in fact, almost always) find this test confusing.

Endocrinology divides naturally into areas based on the major endocrine glands: the pituitary, thyroid, parathyroids, islets of Langerhans, adrenals, ovaries, and testes. In this book each of these areas is detailed in a section consisting of several chapters. In each chapter key concepts are emphasized, and illustrations are used freely. Questions are provided with answers and explanations.

I hope that this review provides a foundation for an understanding of the field of endocrinology, and that the reader will build upon this foundation by reading more detailed references and by learning through clinical experience.

Victor Adlin, M.D.

Acknowledgments

I am grateful to the physicians at Temple University School of Medicine and Temple University Hospital who graciously provided illustrations for this book: I. Bruce Elfenbein, M.D., Kai Ni, M.D., Chik-Kwun Tang, M.D., and Stephen W. Wong, M.D.

Acknowledgements

Contents

The Pituitary Gland

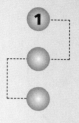

Pituitary Structure and Function

The anterior pituitary gland produces growth hormone and trophic hormones that control the function of the thyroid, adrenals, and gonads. The posterior pituitary gland stores and releases antidiuretic hormone.

ANATOMY

 The pituitary gland is a pea-sized structure in the sella turcica, and is attached to the hypothalamus by the pituitary stalk.

- The anterior pituitary is derived from endodermal structures. The many specific cell types of the anterior pituitary are distinguished by electron microscopy and immunohistochemical staining. Each cell type produces a specific hormone: somatotrophs produce growth hormone; corticotrophs, adrenocorticotropic hormone (ACTH); thyrotrophs, thyroid-stimulating hormone (TSH); gonadotrophs, luteinizing hormone (LH) and follicle-stimulating hormone (FSH); and lactotrophs, prolactin.

- The posterior pituitary is derived from neural ectoderm, and consists mainly of axonal fibers whose cell bodies are in the supraoptic and paraventricular nuclei in the hypothalamus.

- Vasopressin, the antidiuretic hormone, is made in the hypothalamic nuclei. It is packaged in granules and transported down the pituitary stalk to the posterior pituitary, where it is stored and released.

- The hormone oxytocin, which stimulates uterine contraction during delivery, is also made in these hypothalamic nuclei and is handled in the same way as vasopressin.

- A system of portal veins in the pituitary stalk allows hypothalamic hormones to travel down the stalk and reach the anterior pituitary in high concentration, where they stimulate or inhibit the production of pituitary hormones (Fig. 1-1).

1

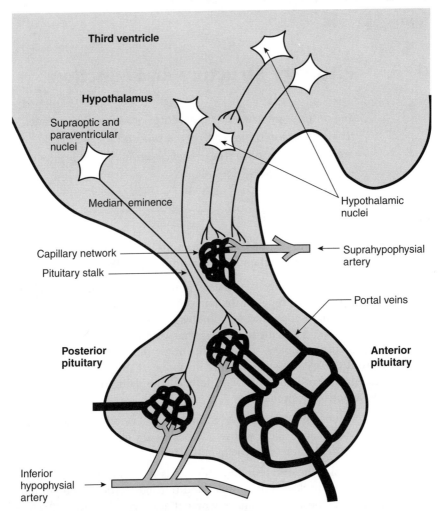

Figure 1-1. The hypothalamic–pituitary axis. Hormones that control pituitary hormone production are synthesized in the hypothalamic nuclei, released in the median eminence, and transported via the capillary network and portal veins to the anterior pituitary.

CONTROL OF PITUITARY HORMONE PRODUCTION AND RELEASE

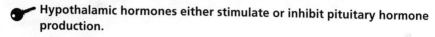 **Hypothalamic hormones either stimulate or inhibit pituitary hormone production.**

- Hypothalamic hormones that *stimulate* the production and release of pituitary hormones include corticotropin-releasing hormone (CRH), thyrotropin-releasing hormone (TRH), gonadotropin-releasing hormone (GnRH), and growth hormone-releasing hormone (GHRH).

- Hypothalamic hormones that *inhibit* pituitary hormone production are dopamine, which is the prolactin-inhibiting factor, and somatostatin, which inhibits GH production.

The target organs of the pituitary (i.e., thyroid, adrenal, gonads) produce hormones that have a negative-feedback effect on the pituitary.

- A negative-feedback effect is seen when increased target-organ hormone levels inhibit pituitary production of the corresponding trophic hormone, and decreased levels stimulate the trophic hormone. Negative-feedback action can affect the hypothalamic hormones in a similar way.

- Release of vasopressin from the posterior pituitary is triggered by nerve impulses originating in the hypothalamus. The main stimuli for these impulses are an increase in plasma osmolality and a decrease in plasma volume.

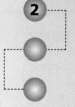

Hypopituitarism

Destruction or functional abnormality of the hypothalamic–pituitary axis leads to a syndrome of multiple hormonal deficits, which can include growth hormone deficiency, hypothyroidism, adrenal insufficiency, hypogonadism, and, if the vasopressin-producing structures are affected, diabetes insipidus.

CAUSES OF HYPOPITUITARISM

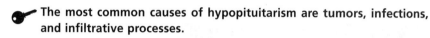 **The most common causes of hypopituitarism are tumors, infections, and infiltrative processes.**

■ Most often, hypopituitarism is caused by tumors of the pituitary or nearby structures, or surgical attempts to remove the tumors.

• Tumors affecting the hypothalamic–pituitary area include pituitary adenomas, craniopharyngiomas, meningiomas, and metastatic tumors. Craniopharyngiomas arise from remnants of Rathke's pouch, an embryologic outpouching of the oral ectoderm from which the anterior pituitary arises; these tumors tend to be suprasellar and to occur early in life.

■ Infectious and infiltrative processes such as sarcoidosis, hemochromatosis, fungal infections, and tuberculosis may also cause hypopituitarism.

■ Pituitary infarction can occur during or after a delivery complicated by a hypotensive episode, (i.e., Sheehan's syndrome) because the pituitary gland is twice its normal size and vulnerable to a sudden decrease in its blood supply at the end of pregnancy. Sheehan's syndrome causes hypopituitarism.

MANIFESTATIONS OF PITUITARY TUMORS

 Pituitary tumors can cause hypopituitarism and neurologic symptoms.

■ Destructive lesions affecting the hypothalamus or pituitary stalk can cause hypopituitarism not only by destroying pituitary tissue, but also by removing the stimulatory effects of hypothalamic factors on pituitary hormone secretion.

- Paradoxically, prolactin levels can rise rather than fall in the presence of a lesion. This occurs because the hypothalamus inhibits prolactin secretion via dopamine (prolactin-inhibiting factor), whereas the hypothalamus stimulates the secretion of other pituitary hormones.

■ In addition to causing hypopituitarism, tumors of the pituitary can cause headaches, other neurologic effects, and optic nerve compression. They can press upward on the inferior surface of the optic chiasm, causing visual loss in the superior temporal quadrants, then bitemporal hemianopsia (Fig. 2-1).

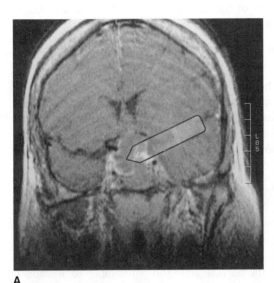

A

Figure 2-1. Magnetic resonance imaging (MRI) studies of the brain show a pituitary macroadenoma in a 50-year-old woman. (*A*) An irregularly shaped lesion (arrow) extends upward from the pituitary fossa into the right cavernous and sphenoid sinuses. The lesion is causing superior displacement of the optic chiasm. (The patient had marked visual impairment.)

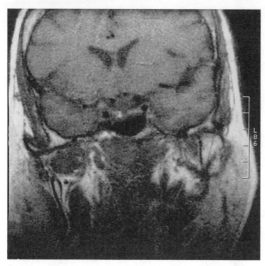

Figure 2-1. Continued (*B*) Much of the tumor was removed surgically, and the patient was treated with bromocriptine and octreotide. (The tumor produced growth hormone and prolactin.) Two years later, little residual tumor can be seen on MRI studies.

B

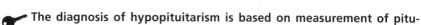

MANIFESTATIONS OF HYPOPITUITARISM

- Growth hormone deficiency leads to growth failure in children. In adults, the effects of growth hormone deficiency are less striking, consisting mainly of changes in body composition (e.g., decreased muscle mass, increased fat mass) and possibly a decrease in strength and exercise capacity.

- Deficiencies of adrenocorticotropic hormone (ACTH), thyroid-stimulating hormone (TSH), luteinizing hormone (LH), and follicle-stimulating hormone (FSH) are considered in Chapters 22 (hypoadrenalism), 8 (hypothyroidism), and 31 (hypogonadism).

- No significant clinical abnormalities result from prolactin deficiency.

DIAGNOSIS OF HYPOPITUITARISM

The diagnosis of hypopituitarism is based on measurement of pituitary hormones and target organ hormones.

- Diagnosis also can require measuring the response of these hormones to stimulation and suppression.

  - For example, growth hormone levels can be undetectable in normal persons; proving that levels are inadequate requires demonstrating a lack of normal response to stimulation by insulin-induced hypoglycemia (Fig. 2-2), or other maneuvers.

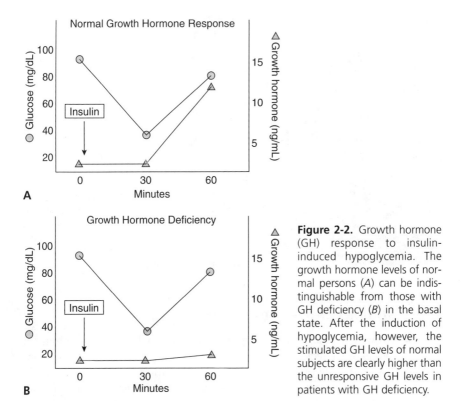

Figure 2-2. Growth hormone (GH) response to insulin-induced hypoglycemia. The growth hormone levels of normal persons (*A*) can be indistinguishable from those with GH deficiency (*B*) in the basal state. After the induction of hypoglycemia, however, the stimulated GH levels of normal subjects are clearly higher than the unresponsive GH levels in patients with GH deficiency.

TREATMENT OF HYPOPITUITARISM

 Goals of treatment are different for children and adults.

- Growth hormone deficiency in children is treated with injections of growth hormone, in an attempt to achieve normal height.

- In adults, it is not yet certain whether the beneficial effects of growth hormone on body composition and possibly other manifestations are worth the economic cost and potential side-effects of growth hormone replacement therapy.

- Replacement therapy with levothyroxine, cortisol, and either estrogen or testosterone is necessary in most adults with hypopituitarism, and with levothyroxine and cortisol in children.

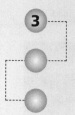

Oversecretion of Pituitary Hormones

3

Pituitary adenomas, depending on their cell type, can produce excessive amounts of growth hormone, prolactin, adrenocorticotropic hormone (ACTH), follicle-stimulating hormone (FSH), luteinizing hormone (LH), or thyroid-stimulating hormone (TSH). Many pituitary adenomas do not produce significant amounts of any hormone.

ACROMEGALY

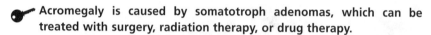 **Acromegaly is caused by somatotroph adenomas, which can be treated with surgery, radiation therapy, or drug therapy.**

- Manifestations of acromegaly (Table 3-1) are the result of excess production of growth hormone by the pituitary adenoma and the resulting excess insulin-like growth factor (IGF-1) production by the liver.

- The diagnosis of acromegaly is suggested by a typical change in the patient's appearance (Fig. 3-1) and the other clinical manifestations.

  - The somatotroph adenoma responsible for the disease may or may not be seen on magnetic resonance imaging (MRI).

Table 3-1. Manifestations of Acromegaly
Skeletal and soft tissue changes

Enlargement of hands (especially fingertips) and feet
  Increased ring, glove, shoe size
Coarsening of facial features
  Thick skinfolds: brow, nasolabial creases
  Enlargement of nose and mandible, with prognathism, spreading of teeth
Enlargement of internal organs: heart, lungs, liver, spleen, kidneys
Skin thickening and interstitial edema, with swelling and firmness of soft tissue
Osteoarthritis
Entrapment neuropathies, especially carpal tunnel syndrome
X-ray changes: enlargement of sinuses, tufting of distal phalanges, cortical thickening

Metabolic changes
Decreased glucose tolerance (anti-insulin actions of growth hormone) Hyperphosphatemia (increased tubular reabsorption of phosphate caused by growth hormone)

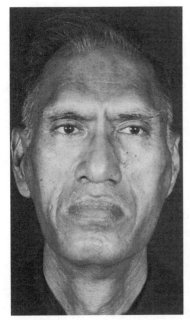 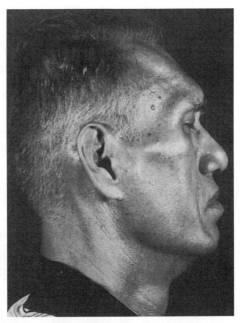

Figure 3-1. These pictures of a man with acromegaly demonstrate prominence of the mandible, zygomatic arches, and supraorbital ridges, and exaggerated skinfolds. (From Merimee TJ and Grant MB: Growth hormone and its disorders, In: BECKER KL: *Principles and Practice of Endocrinology and Metabolism.* Philadelphia, J.B. Lippincott Company, 1990, p. 131.)

- Elevated blood levels of growth hormone and IGF-1 are confirmatory.

- The most sensitive and specific test for acromegaly is the measurement of growth hormone following an oral glucose tolerance test with 75 g of glucose.

  In normal individuals and in patients successfully cured of acromegaly, the growth hormone level will be suppressed to less than 1 ng/mL within 2 hours of glucose ingestion.

■ Transsphenoidal pituitary adenomectomy is performed if the tumor is large.

■ Radiation therapy can be used to treat smaller tumors or residual tumor following surgery; its full effects may not be seen for several years.

■ Acromegaly can be treated pharmacologically with octreotide or bromocriptine.

- Octreotide, an analog of somatostatin, is given by subcutaneous injection several times daily. Octreotide lowers growth hormone and IGF-1 levels in half the cases.

- Bromocriptine, a dopamine agonist taken by mouth, also can decrease growth hormone production, but is effective in fewer cases than octreotide.

GALACTORRHEA–AMENORRHEA SYNDROME

Lactotroph adenomas produce excess prolactin, causing the galactorrhea–amenorrhea syndrome.

■ Milk production results from direct stimulation of breast cells by prolactin; amenorrhea results from actions of prolactin on the hypothalamic–pituitary axis [suppression of gonadotropin-releasing hormone (GnRH), LH, and FSH production] and on the ovary (inhibition of follicle development).

■ Measurement of serum prolactin levels helps to differentiate a pituitary adenoma from nonneoplastic, or "functional," causes of hyperprolactinemia: tumors often raise prolactin levels above 300 ng/mL (normal is less than 25 ng/mL), whereas functional causes seldom raise levels above 100 to 200 ng/mL.

- The main nonneoplastic causes of hyperprolactinemia are drugs that inhibit dopamine activity and thus prevent its normal inhibition of prolactin production. These drugs include psychotropic agents (phenothiazines, butyrophenones, tricyclic antidepressants), antihypertensive drugs (methyldopa, reserpine), metoclopramide, cimetidine, and others.

- Hyperprolactinemia also may be caused by a lesion of the pituitary stalk or hypothalamus that blocks the production of prolactin-inhibiting factor or its transport to the pituitary.

■ Prolactin excess caused by prolactinomas or drugs can be treated with agents that act as dopamine agonists.

- Bromocriptine has been the standard treatment; newer agents include pergolide and cabergoline.

- Dopamine agonists produce a prompt decline in serum prolactin, usually to normal levels, and frequently cause shrinkage of tumor tissue in patients who have not had pituitary surgery or who have residual tumor tissue following surgery.

OTHER SYNDROMES OF PITUITARY HORMONE OVERPRODUCTION

- Pituitary tumors may produce ACTH, causing Cushing's syndrome (see Chapter 23).

- Thyrotroph adenomas that produce TSH are a rare cause of hyperthyroidism; a diagnostic clue is the presence of elevated, rather than suppressed, TSH levels in a hyperthyroid patient.

- FSH and LH secretion by pituitary adenomas is fairly common, but usually does not result in a clear-cut clinical syndrome.

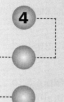

The Posterior Pituitary

Arginine vasopressin, the antidiuretic hormone (ADH), plays an important role in the control of water balance. Inadequate ADH production leads to diabetes insipidus, and excessive ADH causes a syndrome characterized by hyponatremia.

ADH AND WATER BALANCE

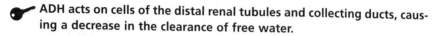 **ADH acts on cells of the distal renal tubules and collecting ducts, causing a decrease in the clearance of free water.**

- ADH binds to receptors on the cell membrane and stimulates adenylate cyclase.

- This action starts a chain of events that increases the permeability of the distal renal tubules and collecting ducts to water.

- Because of the higher osmolality in the renal medulla, water then is reabsorbed from the distal and collecting tubules, decreasing the clearance of free water.

- ADH production in the hypothalamus and release from the posterior pituitary is stimulated by an increase in serum osmolality or a decrease in intravascular volume; the ensuing water retention tends to correct the abnormalities of osmolality, volume, or both.

DIABETES INSIPIDUS

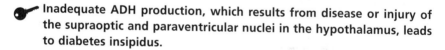 **Inadequate ADH production, which results from disease or injury of the supraoptic and paraventricular nuclei in the hypothalamus, leads to diabetes insipidus.**

- Half the cases of diabetes insipidus are idiopathic; other causes are tumors, surgery, trauma, or infiltrative conditions (e.g., sarcoidosis). Damage to the posterior pituitary does not necessarily lead to diabetes insipidus, provided the hypothalamic nuclei remain intact and able to produce ADH.

- In the absence of adequate ADH, the inability to reabsorb free water and concentrate the urine causes polyuria and thirst. A conscious person with access to water and a normal thirst mechanism is inconvenienced by the polyuria but can maintain hydration; however, an unconscious patient can suffer life-threatening dehydration.

■ Two other causes of hypo-osmolar polyuria must be distinguished from "central" or "neurogenic" diabetes insipidus.

- In *nephrogenic diabetes insipidus,* the renal tubules fail to respond to normal levels of ADH. This may be a congenital abnormality, or may be acquired in association with hypokalemia, hypercalcemia, primary renal disease, or other conditions.

- *Primary polydipsia,* or compulsive water drinking, also may mimic central diabetes insipidus. Serum osmolality tends to be low (255 to 280 mOsm/kg) when increased water intake is the primary abnormality, as in primary polydipsia; serum osmolality is normal or high (280 to 310 mOsm/kg) when loss of free water is the primary abnormality, as in central diabetes insipidus.

■ The water deprivation test is used to distinguish among several causes of hypo-osmolar polyuria.

- Fluid is withheld until urine osmolality, measured hourly, stops increasing (less than 30 mOsm/kg/h for 3 consecutive hours). Serum osmolality is then measured, and 2 μg desmopressin are injected; urine osmolality is measured again in 1 hour.

- The interpretation of this test is shown in Table 4-1.

■ Central diabetes insipidus is most often treated with desmopressin (DDAVP), an analog of arginine vasopressin that is available as oral tablets, nasal spray, or injection.

Table 4-1. Interpretation of the Water Deprivation Test*

	Increase in Urine Osmolality above 280 mOsm/kg with Dehydration	Further Response to ADH
Normal subjects	Yes	No
Diabetes insipidus	No	Yes
Partial diabetes insipidus	Yes	Yes
Nephrogenic diabetes insipidus	No	No

*Normal subjects achieve maximal ADH levels with dehydration, so additional ADH given by injection has no further effect. Central diabetes insipidus is distinguished from nephrogenic diabetes insipidus by the ability of the kidneys to respond to ADH. In patients with partial diabetes insipidus, some concentration of urine can be achieved, but less than maximal ADH can be producded, so there is further urine concentration following administration of exogenous ADH.

SYNDROME OF INAPPROPRIATE ADH SECRETION

🔑 **Hyponatremia characterizes the syndrome of inappropriate ADH secretion (SIADH).**

- Oat-cell lung carcinoma and other tumors may produce ADH.

  - This is an example of ectopic hormone production, that is, production of a hormone by neoplastic tissue derived from cells that do not normally secrete that hormone.

- More common causes of ADH hypersecretion, through unknown mechanisms, are diseases affecting the lungs, central nervous system, and other organs.

- The dominant manifestation of ADH excess is hyponatremia. Water retention sets in motion compensatory mechanisms that minimize the expansion of extracellular fluid volume, but at the expense of dilutional hyponatremia (Fig. 4-1).

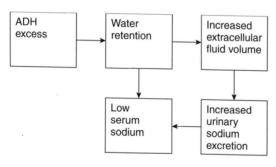

Figure 4-1. The pathophysiology of SIADH. Volume expansion stimulates the urinary excretion of sodium and water, minimizing the volume expansion. Serum sodium concentration, however, is lowered both by the dilution induced by water retention and by the loss of sodium in the urine.

- SIADH is diagnosed when hyponatremia is associated with continued urinary sodium excretion greater than 20 mmol/24 hours, and conditions that might cause *appropriate* increased ADH production are excluded (e.g., adrenal insufficiency, renal disease, cirrhosis, nephrotic syndrome, congestive heart failure).

  - Urinary sodium excretion *less than* 20 mmol/24 hours suggests sodium depletion, rather than water retention, as the primary abnormality.

- The sequence of events shown in Figure 4-1 cannot occur without adequate water intake. Therefore, the primary treatment of SIADH is restricting fluid to 500 to 1000 mL daily.

- If fluid restriction is unsuccessful or cannot be enforced, demeclo-cycline can be given; this antibiotic has the unexpected, but useful, side-effect of antagonizing the action of ADH on renal tubules.

- If hyponatremia is severe, hypertonic saline may have to be given, but its effect is temporary. Serum sodium levels should not be raised faster than 12 mmol/L in 24 hours, or central nervous system damage may occur.

The Thyroid Gland

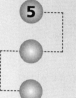

5 Thyroid Physiology

The thyroid regulates metabolism and affects growth and development through the production and release into the circulation of the thyroid hormones—thyroxine and triiodothyronine.

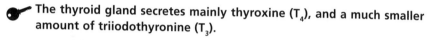

HORMONE PRODUCTION AND RELEASE

🔑 **The thyroid gland secretes mainly thyroxine (T_4), and a much smaller amount of triiodothyronine (T_3).**

- The follicular cells of the thyroid synthesize T_4 and T_3 by trapping and oxidizing circulating iodide, which is followed by the iodination of tyrosyl residues in thyroglobulin. Finally, the coupling of two diiodotyrosine residues forms T_4, whereas the coupling of a diiodotyrosine and a monoiodotyrosine residue forms T_3 (Fig. 5-1).

- T_4 and T_3 are stored in the colloid of the thyroid follicles as part of a large protein molecule, thyroglobulin.

- T_4 and T_3 are released by the processes of endocytosis of thyroglobulin into the follicular cell, cleavage of T_3 and T_4 from thyroglobulin by lysosomal enzymes, and secretion into the bloodstream.

- Thyroid-stimulating hormone (TSH, thyrotropin) binds to receptors on the cell membrane of the thyroid follicular cells (Fig. 5-2). TSH stimulates the synthesis and release of T_4 and T_3, and growth of the thyroid gland.

  - TSH is produced and released by pituitary thyrotroph cells, a process that is regulated by negative feedback from circulating T_4 and T_3.

- About one third of the secreted T_4 is converted to T_3 by monodeiodination in peripheral tissues, primarily the liver. About 20% of circulating T_3 is secreted by the thyroid, and 80% is derived from peripheral conversion of T_4.

17

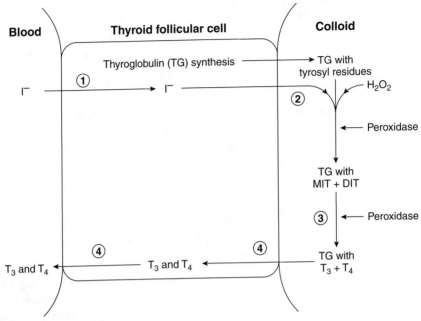

① Trapping of iodide

② Organification of iodide

③ Coupling

④ Secretion (Colloid resorption, proteolysis)

A

Figure 5-1. (*A*) Steps in the production and release of thyroid hormone.

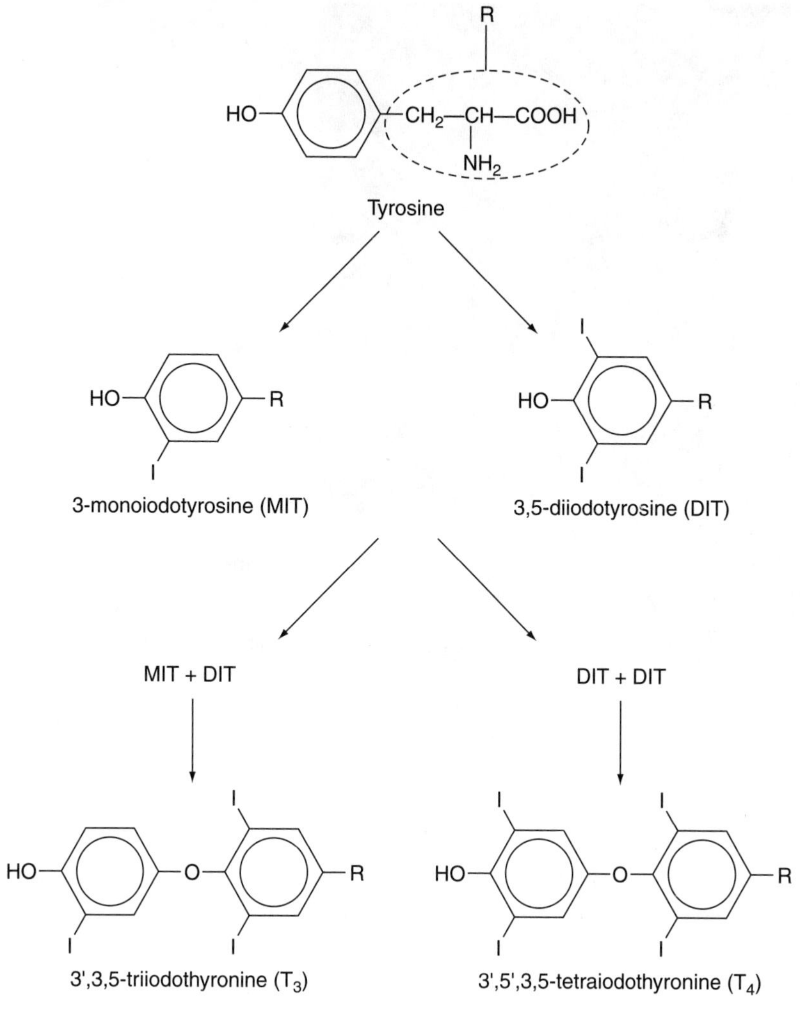

Figure 5-1. (B) Synthesis of T_3 and T_4. (*MIT*, monoiodotyrosine; *DIT*, diiodotyrosine)

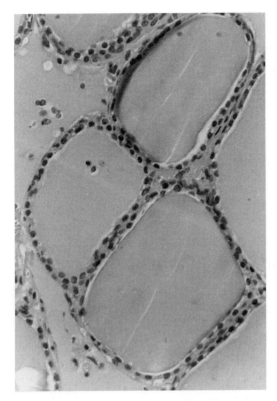

Figure 5-2. Photomicrograph of a normal thyroid gland (original magnification ×40). The thyroid follicles consist of colloid surrounded by a single layer of cuboidal epithelial cells, the thyroid follicular cells. (Courtesy of Chik-Kwun Tang, M.D.)

MODE OF ACTION OF THYROID HORMONE

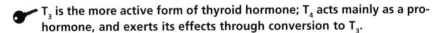 T_3 is the more active form of thyroid hormone; T_4 acts mainly as a prohormone, and exerts its effects through conversion to T_3.

■ Within the cells that are targets of thyroid hormone action, T_3 binds to specific T_3 receptors in the nucleus. These receptors bind to regulatory regions of genes and affect gene expression.

EFFECTS OF THYROID HORMONE

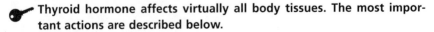 Thyroid hormone affects virtually all body tissues. The most important actions are described below.

■ *Calorigenesis:* Oxygen consumption is increased, with an increase in the rate of energy metabolism and heat production. Increased availability of substrate for energy metabolism (i.e., glucose, fatty acids) results from the carbohydrate and lipid effects of thyroid hormone.

- *Effects on protein metabolism:* Enzymes and other proteins are synthesized more rapidly.

- *Effects on carbohydrate metabolism:* Increases are seen in gastrointestinal absorption of glucose, and in hepatic glucose release, owing to enhanced gluconeogenesis and glycogenolysis. These effects tend to increase glucose availability to the tissues.

- *Effects on lipid metabolism:* Lipid production is increased, but lipid degradation is increased to a greater extent. The result is a decrease in the stores and blood levels of triglycerides, cholesterol, and other lipids. Increased lipolysis makes fatty acids more available as substrate for energy metabolism.

- *Interactions with catecholamines:* Thyroid hormone produces physiologic changes (e.g., tachycardia, sweating, and lipolysis) that are similar to changes that occur with increased sympathetic nervous system activity. These changes are caused by increased sensitivity to catecholamines, apparently mediated by increased catecholamine receptors and postreceptor sensitivity, rather than by changes in blood epinephrine or norepinephrine levels.

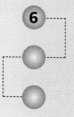

Thyroid Function Tests

Thyroid function is evaluated by measuring circulating levels of thyroxine (T_4), triiodothyronine (T_3), and thyroid-stimulating hormone (TSH). In addition, measurements of the uptake of radioiodine by the thyroid gland, and indirect indicators of the status of serum thyroid-hormone binding proteins are used to evaluate thyroid function.

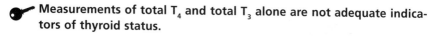

BLOOD LEVELS OF T_4 AND T_3

🗝 **Measurements of total T_4 and total T_3 alone are not adequate indicators of thyroid status.**

- About 99.95% of circulating T_4 is bound to thyroid-hormone binding proteins (thyroxine-binding globulin, thyroxine-binding prealbumin, and albumin). The 0.05% that is free, however, is the physiologically important fraction.

  - If the level of binding proteins is altered, the total T_4 concentration (bound plus free), which is commonly measured as the serum T_4, may not reflect the level of free T_4.

  - The same considerations are true for T_3.

- Several conditions can raise or lower the concentrations of thyroid-hormone binding protein (THBP) (Table 6-1). The hypothalamic–pituitary–thyroid feedback mechanism maintains the free T_4 and free T_3 concentrations in the normal range, so patients with these conditions remain euthyroid. But an increased total T_4 level is needed to maintain a normal free T_4 level if binding proteins are increased, as in

Table 6-1. Conditions That Alter the Levels of Thyroid-Hormone Binding Proteins

Increased THBP	Decreased THBP
Pregnancy	Androgens, anabolic steroid therapy
Estrogen therapy (e.g., oral contraceptives, postmenopausal estrogen replacement)	Hypoproteinemia (e.g., malnutrition, nephrotic syndrome)
Genetic thyroxine-binding globulin excess	Genetic thyroxine-binding globulin deficiency
Hepatic disease	Hepatic disease

a woman who is pregnant or taking estrogens. Conversely, a low total T_4 but normal free T_4 is present in a person with decreased THBP.

- ■ Because the total T_4 measurement alone is an inadequate indicator of thyroid status, either free T_4 itself must be measured, or a free T_4 index may be calculated by using an indirect estimate of hormone binding, such as the T_3-resin uptake along with the total T_4.

  - • The T_3-resin uptake (T-uptake) measures the unoccupied binding sites on THBP (Fig. 6-1). Radiolabeled T_3 competitively binds to

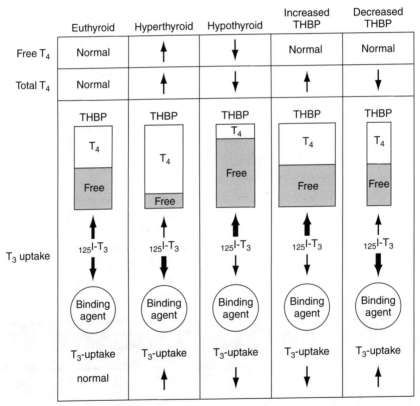

Figure 6-1. Changes in thyroid function tests with hyperthyroidism, hypothyroidism, and alterations in thyroid-hormone binding proteins (THBP). In the bar representing THBP, "free" indicates the relative number of unoccupied binding sites for thyroid hormone. The percent T_3 uptake is determined by counting the radiolabeled T_3 attached to the binding agent.

the patient's thyroid-binding proteins or to a solid binding agent such as a resin, and the percent bound to the resin is determined.

> In hyperthyroidism (unchanged proteins, increased thyroid hormone), there are fewer unoccupied binding sites on the proteins, so the resin uptake is increased.

> In hypothyroidism (unchanged proteins, decreased thyroid hormone), there are more unoccupied sites on the proteins, so the resin uptake is decreased.

- Thus, in hyperthyroidism the total T_4 and T_3 uptake are both elevated and in hypothyroidism they are both decreased. But in euthyroid individuals with altered THBP, the total T_4 and T_3 uptake are altered in opposite directions (see Fig. 6-1).

- Therefore, the ratio of observed-to-expected T_3 uptake, if applied as a correction factor to the total T_4, will alter the T_4 toward normal if an abnormality of binding proteins is the problem, but will exaggerate the increase or decrease in total T_4 if the patient has hyperthyroidism or hypothyroidism. This calculated value is called the free T_4 index (Fig. 6-2).

Formula: $\dfrac{T_3\ \text{Uptake}}{\text{Normal } T_3\ \text{Uptake}} \times \text{Total } T_4 \quad = \quad$ Free T_4 Index (Normal range same as for total T_4)

Case: Slightly hyperthyroid-appearing woman taking estrogen has total T_4 of 16.0 µg/dL (normal: 4.5–12.5).

Scenario 1: $T_4 = 16.0$ µg/dL
T_3 uptake = 40% (normal: 25–35)

Free T_4 index = $\dfrac{40}{30} \times 16.0 = 21.3$ (high)

Conclusion: Patient is hyperthyroid.

Scenario 2: $T_4 = 16.0$ µg/dL
T_3 uptake = 15%

Free T_4 index = $\dfrac{15}{30} \times 16.0 = 8.0$ (normal)

Conclusion: Patient is euthyroid; elevated total T4 is caused by estrogen.

Figure 6-2. Calculation of free T_4 index.

- Serum total T_3 (also referred to as T3-RIA (radioimmunoassay)—*not* to be confused with the T_3 resin uptake—is a less sensitive indicator of hypothyroidism, and frequently falls below normal as a nonspecific response to nonthyroidal illness or undernutrition.

  - For these reasons, the free T_4 or free T_4 index is generally more useful as an indicator of thyroid hormone status. In a clinically hyperthyroid patient with lowered TSH but normal free T_4 and free T_4 index, however, the total T_3 (along with the T_3 resin uptake) or the free T3 must be measured to rule out T_3-toxicosis, in which only T_3 is abnormally increased in the circulation.

SERUM TSH

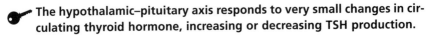 **The hypothalamic–pituitary axis responds to very small changes in circulating thyroid hormone, increasing or decreasing TSH production.**

- Serum TSH may be elevated in hypothyroidism or lowered in hyperthyroidism when the serum thyroid hormone levels have changed only slightly and are still in the normal range. For this reason, the serum TSH level is the most useful screening test for hyperthyroidism or primary hypothyroidism.

- In secondary hypothyroidism caused by inadequate pituitary production of TSH, the serum TSH level is not useful in evaluating thyroid function and the free T_4 or free T_4 index must be relied on.

RADIOIODINE STUDIES

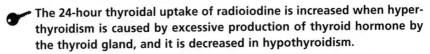 **The 24-hour thyroidal uptake of radioiodine is increased when hyperthyroidism is caused by excessive production of thyroid hormone by the thyroid gland, and it is decreased in hypothyroidism.**

- Radioiodine uptake measurement is most useful when less common causes of hyperthyroidism, *not* caused by increased thyroid gland production of hormone, must be ruled out. In such cases serum thyroid hormone levels are elevated, and serum TSH is decreased, but radioiodine uptake is *decreased* rather than elevated.

  - *Subacute thyroiditis:* Thyroid hormone is released into the circulation because of injury to the gland. Radioiodine uptake is decreased because the thyroid cells are injured and because TSH is suppressed by the increased thyroid hormone level.

- *Thyrotoxicosis factitia* or other cause of excessive ingestion of thyroid hormone: TSH is suppressed, endogenous hormone production is decreased, and so radioiodine uptake is low.

■ A scintiscan of the thyroid, done in conjunction with the 24-hour uptake measurement, indicates areas of the gland with increased or decreased function.

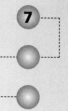

Autoimmune Thyroid Disease

Autoimmune disease affecting the thyroid gland may lead to inflammation and enlargement of the gland, hypothyroidism, or hyperthyroidism.

MECHANISMS OF THYROID AUTOIMMUNITY

- Factors involved in the development of thyroid autoimmuinity are genetic differences (e.g., variation in expression of major histocompatibility complex antigens by thyroid cells); endogenous factors (e.g., estrogen or other hormone levels); and environmental factors (e.g., infection, stress).

- Thyroid autoimmunity may start with the production of interferon gamma by intrathyroidal T cells, which causes thyroid follicular cells to express major histocompatibility complex class II molecules.

- Thyroid cells then present thyroid antigens to the T cells, starting the autoimmune process. The main thyroid autoantigens include thyroglobulin, thyroid peroxidase, and the thyroid-stimulating hormone (TSH) receptor.

MECHANISMS IN AUTOIMMUNE HYPOTHYROIDISM AND HASHIMOTO'S THYROIDITIS

- Cytotoxicity is caused by $CD8^+$ T cells that infiltrate the thyroid gland. Intrathyroidal T cells release cytokines (including interleukin 1, interleukin 6, tumor necrosis factor, and interferon gamma) that impair thyroid cell function, causing autoimmune hypothyroidism.

- Autoantibodies to thyroid peroxidase (which is the enzyme that catalyzes the iodination of tyrosine residues of thyroglobulin) (Fig. 5-1A) and antibodies to other antigens activate compliment, producing damage to thyroid cells.

MECHANISMS IN GRAVES' DISEASE

- Antibodies to the TSH receptor may bind to the receptor and act like TSH, stimulating adenylate cyclase and causing increased thyroid hormone production and growth of thyroid cells (Fig. 7-1).

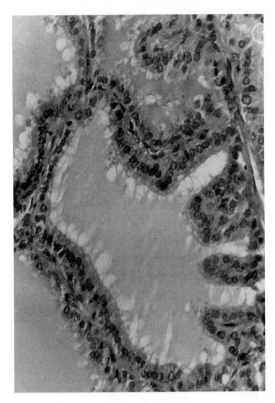

Figure 7-1. Photomicrograph of the thyroid of a patient with Graves' disease (original magnification ×40). Hyperplasia of the thyroid follicular cells and papillary infolding are visible. (Courtesy of Chik-Kwun Tang, M.D.)

- Many of the immune events noted in Hashimoto's thyroiditis also occur in Graves' disease.

  - This may explain the late occurrence of hypothyroidism sometimes seen in Graves' disease, even when antithyroid drugs rather than ablative therapy (i.e., surgery or radioiodine) were used to treat the hyperthyroidism, and the occasional overlapping manifestations of more than one autoimmune thyroid disease in a single patient.

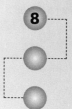

Hypothyroidism

Inadequate circulating levels of thyroid hormone produce a state of decreased metabolic function, with manifestations in all major body systems.

CAUSES OF HYPOTHYROIDISM

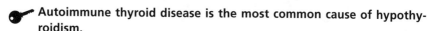

Autoimmune thyroid disease is the most common cause of hypothyroidism.

- Hashimoto's thyroiditis (chronic autoimmune thyroiditis) usually presents with thyroid enlargement. The patient may be hypothyroid when the disease is first diagnosed, may become hypothyroid later, or may remain euthyroid.

  - Thyroid enlargement is caused by inflammatory changes in the gland, with lymphocytic infiltration the predominant histologic finding, and perhaps by thyroid-stimulating hormone (TSH) acting on thyroid cells when hormone production becomes inadequate (Figs. 8-1 and 8-2).

  - Idiopathic atrophy of the thyroid, a common form of hypothyroidism, is probably an atrophic form of Hashimoto's thyroiditis.

- Hypothyroidism frequently occurs following the treatment of Graves' disease, sometimes many years later. Presumed causes are removal or destruction of thyroid tissue by surgery or radioiodine, and the presence of destructive antibodies in addition to the stimulatory antithyroid antibodies that caused the Graves' disease.

- Secondary hypothyroidism is a prominent finding in panhypopituitarism.

- Iodine deficiency has been eliminated in most developed countries, but remains an important cause of hypothyroidism in some areas of the world.

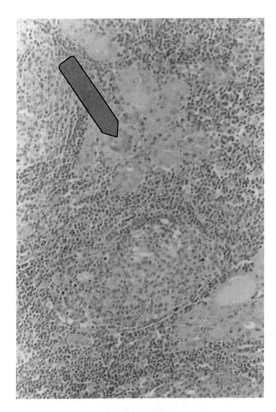

Figure 8-1. Photomicrograph of thyroid of a patient with chronic autoimmune thyroiditis (original magnification ×20). There is atrophy of the thyroid follicles, and dense infiltration by lymphocytes with germinal centers and plasma cells. The oncocytic appearance of many follicular cells (*arrow*) is characterized by increased cell size and acidophilic cytoplasm. (Courtesy of Chik-Kwun Tang, M.D.)

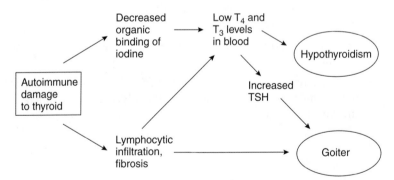

Figure 8-2. Pathogenesis of chronic autoimmune thyroiditis.

Table 8-1. Manifestations of Hypothyroidism

Symptoms	Physical Findings	Additional Effects on Organ Systems
Weakness, lethargy, fatigue	Thickened, puffy features (eyelids, face, hands)	Cardiovascular: decrease in cardiac output; pericardial effusion
Dry skin, coarse hair	Yellowish, dry skin	
Cold intolerance		Respiratory: hypoventilation; pleural effusion
Constipation	Loss of lateral portion of eyebrows	
Weight gain	Nonpitting edema	Nervous system: decreased mental function; depression, other psychiatric changes
Hoarseness	Hypothermia	
Menorrhagia	Bradycardia	
Hearing loss	Slow return of deep tendon reflexes	Blood: normochromic normocytic anemia

MANIFESTATIONS OF HYPOTHYROIDISM

■ Abnormalities result from the decreased rate of energy metabolism, and the accumulation of mucinous mucopolysaccharide-rich material in many tissues (Table 8-1, Fig. 8-3).

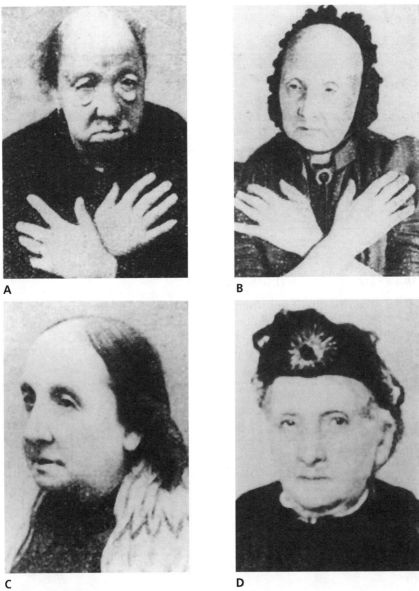

Figure 8-3. Severe hypothyroidism (myxedema). This patient was first reported in 1894, long before early detection was made possible by sensitive blood hormone measurements. (*A*) The patient at approximately age 60, before treatment. Symptoms of hypothyroidism had been present for 20 years. Hair loss and thickening and puffiness of the eyelids, lips, and face are evident. The patient was bedridden and mentally impaired. (*B*) After 5 weeks' treatment with thyroid extract. (*C*) After 15 months' treatment. The patient eventually became physically active and mentally competent. (*D*) Shortly before her death at age 94 in 1924. (Reproduced with permission from Raven HM: The life-history of a case of myxoedema. *Brit Med J* 2:622, 1924.)

DIAGNOSIS OF HYPOTHYROIDISM

 Elevation of the TSH level is the most sensitive indicator of hypothy-roidism; however, any of the manifestations listed in Table 8-1 should trigger a screening test, even though some may be misconstrued as normal changes of aging (e.g., fatigue, constipation, weight gain, cognitive changes).

■ Hypothyroidism is common in the elderly, especially in women (5% to 10% prevalence in many series); therefore, screening with TSH measurement every few years is prudent.

■ As thyroid function begins to falter, a slight fall in blood levels of thyroid hormone triggers a disproportionate increase in TSH production; that is, TSH levels become elevated at an early stage in thyroid failure, when thyroid hormone levels may still be in the normal range (although below their original concentration) (Fig. 8-4). TSH elevation, therefore, is the most sensitive indicator of hypothyroidism.

■ The diagnosis of hypothyroidism is confirmed by the finding of decreased levels of free thyroxine (T_4) or the free T_4 index.

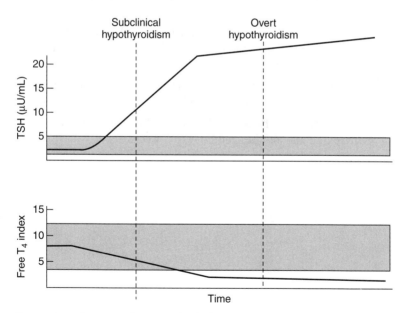

Figure 8-4. Changes in hormone levels during the development of hypothyroidism. The blood TSH level becomes elevated before the free T_4 index has fallen below the normal range.

TREATMENT OF HYPOTHYROIDISM

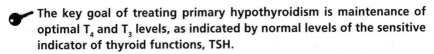 **The key goal of treating primary hypothyroidism is maintenance of optimal T_4 and T_3 levels, as indicated by normal levels of the sensitive indicator of thyroid functions, TSH.**

- L-thyroxine (Synthroid, Levothroid, Levoxyl) is the recommended treatment for hypothyroidism. T_4 has a long half-life (7 to 8 days) and is gradually transformed to triiodothyronine (T_3) in peripheral tissues; therefore, its use results in fairly constant blood levels of both T_4 and T_3 in approximately the normal ratio. Although T_3 and combinations of T_3 and T_4 are available, T_3 has a short half-life and, unless taken in multiple daily doses, would result in widely fluctuating blood levels.

- The usual range of T_4 doses needed to treat hypothyroidism is 50 to 200 μg once daily. An initial dose of 50 μg may be raised at 2- to 3-week intervals. Patients who are elderly or fragile, or those who have cardiac disease, should receive a lower initial dose and more gradual increases.

- Treatment is aimed at maintaining the serum TSH level in the normal range.

  - A low TSH level indicates that overtreatment has caused subclinical hyperthyroidism, which may have undesired long-term effects on bone density and cardiac function.

  - Symptoms that persist when TSH has been brought into the mid-normal range are unlikely to be related to thyroid disfunction.

  - The full effect on the serum TSH level of a change in the dose of L-thyroxine may not be seen for 4 to 6 weeks.

SUBCLINICAL HYPOTHYROIDISM

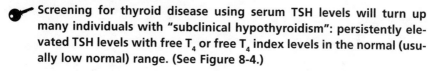 **Screening for thyroid disease using serum TSH levels will turn up many individuals with "subclinical hypothyroidism": persistently elevated TSH levels with free T_4 or free T_4 index levels in the normal (usually low normal) range. (See Figure 8-4.)**

- Persons with subclinical hypothyroidism are more likely than unaffected persons to have mild manifestations of hypothyroidism, including slightly higher levels of LDL cholesterol.

  - Overt hypothyroidism (decreased free T_4 or free T_4 index and increased TSH) develops in about 5% of these individuals each year; this incidence is closer to 20% per year in elderly patients with high titers of antithyroid antibodies.

- Persons with subclinical hypothyroidism probably should be treated if their TSH level is substantially elevated (greater than 10 to 15 mIU/L), if they have symptoms that might be related to hypothyroidism, or if they have elevated antithyroid antibody titers.

  - Lower-than-usual doses of L-thyroxine (25 to 50 μg daily) may be all that is needed to lower the serum TSH level into the normal range.

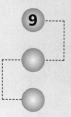

Hyperthyroidism

Excessive circulating levels of thyroid hormone produce a state of increased metabolic function and adrenergic hyperresponsiveness, with effects on all major body systems.

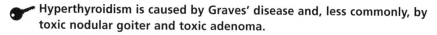

CAUSES OF HYPERTHYROIDISM

Hyperthyroidism is caused by Graves' disease and, less commonly, by toxic nodular goiter and toxic adenoma.

- Graves' disease (diffuse toxic goiter) is the most common cause of hyperthyroidism (Fig. 9-1).

- Much less common than Graves' disease, and affecting mainly older patients, are toxic nodular goiter (Plummer's disease) and toxic adenoma.

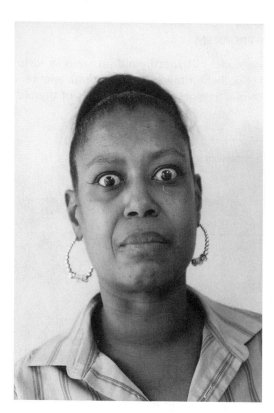

Figure 9-1. A patient showing the typical appearance of Graves' disease, with enlargement of the thyroid gland, and the staring expression caused by exophthalmos and retraction of the upper eyelids.

- In these conditions, one or more areas of the thyroid develop autonomous function and produce excessive amounts of thyroid hormone despite suppression of pituitary thyroid-stimulating hormone (TSH) production.

- In some cases, autonomously functioning nodules have been found to contain cells of a common clonal origin with a somatic mutation of the TSH receptor that causes continuous activation of adenylate cyclase in the absence of TSH (known as a gain-of-function mutation).

■ Subacute thyroiditis may cause a self-limited form of hyperthyroidism[1] due to release of thyroxine (T_4) and triiodothyronine (T_3) from injured thyroid cells.

- A presumed viral form of subacute thyroiditis causes enlargement, pain, and tenderness of the gland.

- An autoimmune form causes a "painless" subacute thyroiditis that is especially common in women during the postpartum period.

MANIFESTATIONS OF HYPERTHYROIDISM

The principal signs and symptoms of hyperthyroidism are related to increased heat production (e.g., heat intolerance, sweating), adrenergic sensitivity (e.g., tachycardia, tremor), and other effects of thyroid hormone (Table 9-1).

■ Several ophthalmic effects may occur with hyperthyroidism.

- Upper lid retraction, causing stare and lid lag, may occur in any form of hyperthyroidism.

Table 9-1. Manifestations of Graves' Disease

Symptoms	Signs	Eye Manifestations
Weight loss	Thyroid enlargement, bruit	Proptosis
Weakness, fatigue	Tachycardia	Inflammation of conjunctivae, tearing, pain, irritation
Nervousness, irritability	Tremor	
Palpitations	Warm, moist skin	Extraocular movement abnormalities, diplopia
Sweating	Hyperkinesis	
Heat intolerance	Widened pulse pressure	Visual loss
Increased bowel movements	Arrhythmias (atrial fibrillation, premature beats)	

[1]More properly called thyrotoxicosis since increased synthesis of hormone by the thyroid gland is not present.

- Thyroid exophthalmos is thought to be caused by cross reaction of antigens in the orbit with thyroid-specific immune cells and antibodies. It occurs only with Graves' disease and causes significant morbidity only in a minority of patients.

   Inflammatory changes occur in the orbit, with edema due to obstruction of venous drainage, production of glycosaminoglycans by orbital fibroblasts, and swelling of the extraocular muscles and other tissues (Fig. 9-2).

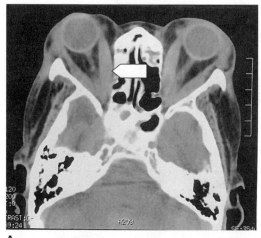

A

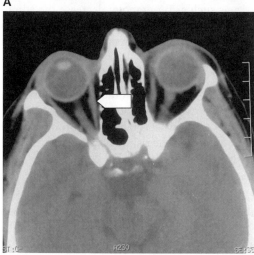

B

Figure 9-2. Computed tomographic (CT) scan of the orbit in a 72-year-old woman with severe Graves' ophthalmopathy. Exophthalmos and swelling of the extraocular muscles (*arrows*) are visible in the patient (*A*) compared with a normal woman (*B*).

- Thyroid storm is a marked exacerbation of the manifestations of hyperthyroidism, usually occurring during an intercurrent stress such as acute nonthyroidal illness, thyroidectomy or other surgery, or delivery.

  • Fever, very severe tachycardia, and delirium are frequently present, and mortality is high.

  • Thyroid storm is probably caused by an acute increase in the fraction of free thyroid hormone, which may occur with severe nonthyroidal illness.

DIAGNOSIS OF HYPERTHYROIDISM

- Hyperthyroidism is suggested by the findings listed in Table 9-1.

- The diagnosis is confirmed by an elevated free T_4 level or free T_4 index, associated with a low serum TSH. The free T3 and free T3 index are also elevated in most cases, although occasionally only one of the two forms of thyroid hormone is elevated. An elevated radioiodine uptake is also present.

TREATMENT OF HYPERTHYROIDISM

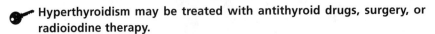 **Hyperthyroidism may be treated with antithyroid drugs, surgery, or radioiodine therapy.**

- β-Adrenergic blocking drugs such as propranolol decrease the adrenergic manifestations (e.g., tachycardia) of hyperthyroidism. They do not affect thyroid function, but may relieve symptoms until thyroid hormone levels can be returned to normal.

- Three definitive methods of treating Graves' disease are available: antithyroid drugs, radioiodine, and surgery (Table 9-2). None can immediately lower the elevated thyroid hormone levels, because even thyroidectomy must be preceded by several weeks or months of antithyroid drug treatment to prevent the risk of perioperative thyroid storm.

  • Antithyroid drugs decrease the synthesis of thyroid hormone by inhibiting the oxidation of iodide and the coupling of iodotyrosines. Although this action occurs promptly, thyroid hormone levels may not become normal for several weeks or months because thyroid hormone already stored in thyroglobulin continues to be released into the circulation.

Table 9-2. Definitive Methods of Treatment of Graves' Disease

Treatment	Advantages	Disadvantages
Antithyroid drugs	Avoid surgery or thyroid ablation	Long-lasting remission in only half of cases
	Avoid hospitalization	Requires greater patient adherence than other methods
	Less post-treatment hypothyroidism	
		Risk of agranulocytosis, other side-effects
Subtotal thyroidectomy	Cure is rapid (but only after weeks of preparation with antithyroid drugs)	Usually requires hospitalization
		Surgical and anesthetic risk
	Shorter period of patient adherence needed than with antithyroid drug therapy	Surgical complications include hypoparathyroidism and recurrent laryngeal nerve paralysis
	Only way to remove a large goiter	
Radioiodine therapy	Avoid hospitalization, surgical and anesthetic risks	Post-treatment hypothyroidism common
	Cure rate approaches 100%	Some patients fear radiation
	Requires least amount of patient adherence	Radiation precautions necessary

- About half of the patients with Graves' disease will have a long-lasting or permanent remission after 1 to 1.5 years' treatment with antithyroid drugs; the reason is unclear.

    Methimazole (Tapazole) or propylthiouracil (PTU) is given until thyroid hormone levels are normal, and then the dose is lowered to about one-third the initial dose and adjusted to maintain euthyroidism for 1 to 1.5 years. Tapazole has the advantage over PTU of being effective in a single daily dose, greatly increasing compliance.

    Minor side effects include skin rash, and are sometimes relieved by switching to the alternative antithyroid drug.

    The main risk of these drugs, however, is agranulocytosis, which occurs in less than 0.5% of patients but is life threatening. To detect this complication as early as possible, patients are instructed to have a complete blood count done immediately if they develop unexplained fever, mouth sores, or a sore throat, and not to resume the medication until a normal white blood cell count is reported.

- Subtotal thyroidectomy is appropriate for patients with very large goiters. It may be the only definitive treatment possible in patients who refuse radioiodine and do not have a long-lasting remission after medical therapy.

- Radioiodine therapy is the treatment of choice of most endocrinologists in the United States for most patients. A single dose of radioiodine will cure the majority of patients within 3 months; a second dose may be given after 3 months if necessary.

■ When treatment of hyperthyroidism is urgent, as in thyroid storm, iodine treatment is used along with antithyroid drugs, β-adrenergic blockers, and supportive measures.

- Iodine, unlike antithyroid drugs, blocks the release of T_4 and T_3 from the thyroid gland, so that the circulating levels of thyroid hormone may fall within 24 hours. Iodine may be given orally as potassium iodide or intravenously as sodium iodide.

- Iodine is not useful in the long-term treatment of Graves' disease because its effect on thyroid hormone release may not last more than several weeks.

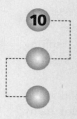

Thyroid Nodules, Thyroid Cancer, and Goiter

10

Enlargement of all or part of the thyroid gland may be caused by benign or malignant disease. Nonmalignant enlargement may cause discomfort and dysfunction through local pressure effects.

APPROACH TO THE PATIENT WITH GOITER OR NODULAR DISEASE

- Enlargement of the thyroid gland may be caused by Graves' disease or nodular toxic goiter, by chronic thyroiditis (with or without hypothyroidism), by iodine deficiency, or by thyroid cancer. Often there is no apparent cause.

- The approach to the patient presenting with goiter requires three main considerations: (1) Does the patient have hyperthyroidism or hypothyroidism? (2) Is thyroid cancer present? (3) Is the goiter causing symptoms by compressing surrounding structures?

THYROID CANCER

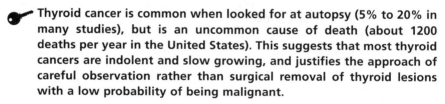

Thyroid cancer is common when looked for at autopsy (5% to 20% in many studies), but is an uncommon cause of death (about 1200 deaths per year in the United States). This suggests that most thyroid cancers are indolent and slow growing, and justifies the approach of careful observation rather than surgical removal of thyroid lesions with a low probability of being malignant.

- Most thyroid cancers are differentiated.
  - Papillary carcinoma makes up about 80% and follicular carcinoma 10% of all thyroid cancers. These tend to be slow-growing, with low mortality rates.
  - Medullary carcinoma, which constitutes 5% of thyroid cancers, has a less favorable prognosis. Anaplastic carcinoma is highly malignant, and makes up about 5% of thyroid cancers.

- Thyroid cancer is treated according to the following principles.
  - The tumor is surgically resected, usually with total or near-total thyroidectomy.

45

- Postoperatively scan for residual tumor capable of trapping radioiodine. This is followed by attempts to destroy any residual tumor with very large doses of radioiodine.

- Levothyroxine is required for lifelong suppression of thyroid-stimulating hormone (TSH), which is a growth factor for many thyroid cancers.

MANAGEMENT OF THYROID NODULES

Thyroid cancer is present in about 5% of solitary thyroid nodules, and dominant hypofunctioning areas in multinodular goiter also must be suspected of malignancy. (Cancer is almost always hypofunctioning on scintiscan, but so are most benign nodules, so this finding is not very helpful.)

- Fine needle aspiration biopsy is the first step in evaluating thyroid nodules; most are benign and can be managed with careful observation rather than surgery (Figs. 10-1 and 10-2).

  - It has been common practice to treat nodules that are presumed benign with "suppressive therapy" with levothyroxine: suppression of TSH presumably may cause nodules to shrink or at least not to grow further. Recent studies, however, suggest that shrinkage occcurs in fewer than one third of nodules, usually the smaller ones. Also, suppression of TSH produces at least a slight degree of subclinical hyperthyroidism, with possible risks to the bones and heart. A reasonable approach would be a trial of suppressive therapy for 6 to 12 months, with continuation only if the nodule shrinks.

- A nodule that is not surgically removed should be observed carefully. Further growth, especially during suppressive therapy, dictates prompt removal of the nodule. Suspected changes in nodule size are confirmed easily by obtaining a baseline ultrasound scan of the thyroid and repeating this study as necessary.

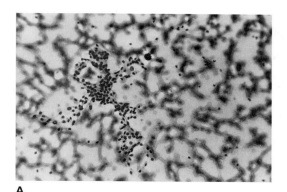

A

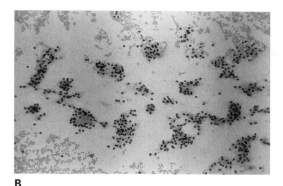

B

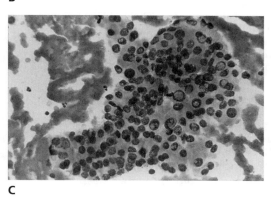

C

Figure 10-1. Fine-needle aspiration biopsy specimens of thyroid nodules. (*A*) No malignancy. Abundant colloid and unremarkable follicular cells suggest a colloid nodular goiter. (*B*) An indeterminant or suspicious sample. The specimen is cellular, with follicular cells in microfollicular formation. There is blood, but no colloid, and atypical cytology. A follicular neoplasm (which could be either an adenoma or a carcinoma) must be ruled out. (*C*) Malignancy. The slide suggests papillary thyroid carcinoma, with nuclear inclusions and papillary fronds. (Courtesy of Kai Ni, M.D.)

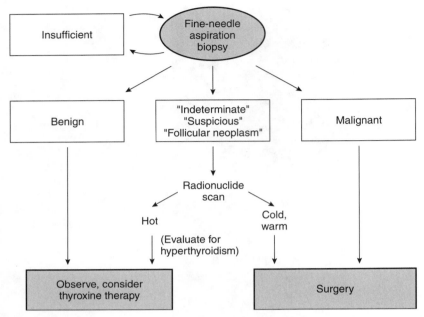

Figure 10-2. Algorithm for evaluation and management of patients with a thyroid nodule. Malignant tumor is found on fine-needle aspiration biopsy in about 5% of cases, indeterminate findings in about 20% and benign nodule in about 75%. The chances of malignancy are less than 5% in a "benign" specimen, about 20% in a "suspicious" specimen, and 97% to 99% in a "malignant" specimen. "Cold," "warm," and "hot" radionuclide scan results refer to radionuclide uptake of the nodule that is less than, equal to, or greater than the uptake by the patient's normal thyroid tissue. (Adapted from: Mazzaferri EL: Management of a solitary thyroid nodule. *N Engl J Med* 328:553–559, 1993; and Singer PA, Cooper DS, Daniels GH, et al: Treatment guidelines for patients with thyroid nodules and well-differentiated thyroid cancer. *Arch Intern Med* 156:2165–2172, 1996.)

MANAGEMENT OF BENIGN GOITER

 Thyroid enlargement can cause choking, neck discomfort, dysphagia, or respiratory obstruction. Tracheal narrowing may be seen on computed tomographic scans of the thyroid in severe cases.

■ Drug therapy, surgery, and radioiodine therapy are all approaches to management of benign goiter.

- Levothyroxine can be administered to suppress TSH in an attempt to decrease the size of a goiter, or at least inhibit further growth.

- If the goiter grows despite suppressive therapy, or if symptoms are unrelieved, it should be surgically removed. Radioiodine therapy may shrink most goiters, and may be considered as an alternative to surgery.

The Parathyroid Glands and Bone Disorders

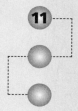

Calcium Homeostasis

Serum calcium has important effects on many body tissues. Its concentration is closely regulated by a system that includes the intestines, bones, kidneys, and several calcium-regulating hormones.

Ionized calcium is the active fraction of serum calcium, which mediates its biological actions and its feedback effects on parathyroid hormone and calcitonin.

- About half the circulating serum calcium exists as ionized calcium, which is the biologically active fraction.

  - Most of the remaining calcium is bound to protein, mainly albumin. A small portion exists as a complex with organic anions such as citrate and bicarbonate.

  - Ionized calcium has important effects on neuromuscular function, on the clotting mechanism, and on the function of enzymes and other proteins in virtually all body tissues. Figure 11-1 summarizes the factors that regulate calcium balance and calcium flux among body compartments.

- Parathyroid hormone (PTH) is an 84-amino acid polypeptide produced by the chief cells of the parathyroid glands. Its biologic activity resides in the N-terminal first 34 amino acids.

  - PTH secretion is controlled by circulating ionized calcium: calcium-sensing receptors on the plasma membranes of parathyroid gland cells detect the level of calcium ion, stimulating PTH secretion if Ca^{2+} is low and inhibiting secretion if Ca^{2+} is high.

  - PTH increases serum calcium by three mechanisms: (1) stimulation of bone resorption, with release of calcium and phosphate into the circulation; (2) increased production of $1,25\text{-}(OH)_2$ vitamin D, which increases intestinal absorption of calcium; and (3) increased

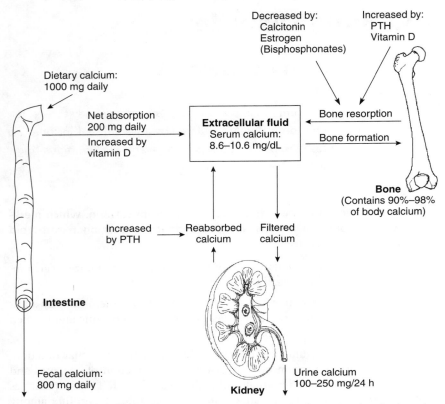

Figure 11-1. Calcium homeostasis. The normal fluxes of calcium involve the intestine, bone, kidneys, and extracellular fluid, and the effects of calciotropic hormones (PTH, vitamin D, calcitonin, estrogen) and medications (bisphosphonates).

reabsorption of filtered calcium and decreased reabsorption of phosphate by the renal tubules.

- Increased phosphaturia raises serum calcium levels because of an inverse relation between serum calcium and phosphate: increased serum concentration of either Ca^{2+} or PO_4 ions raises the calcium–phosphate product, increasing precipitation of calcium phosphate in bone and soft tissues, and lowers the serum concentration of the other ion.

- PTH exerts its effects in bone and kidney mainly by binding to cell-surface receptors and activating the adenylate cyclase–cyclic adenocine monophosphate (cAMP) mechanism.

■ Vitamin D consists of vitamin D_2 (ergocalciferol), from synthetic sources, and D_3 (cholecalciferol), produced in the skin and ingested from animal sources.

- Vitamin D is a prohormone; its metabolism to the active form, 1,25-$(OH)_2$ vitamin D (calcitriol) is shown in Figure 11-2.

- Calcitriol's main actions are to increase the absorption of calcium and phosphate in the intestine, and to increase bone resorption.

■ Calcitonin is a 32-amino acid polypeptide produced by the parafollicular cells (C-cells) of the thyroid gland. It acts directly on osteoclasts to decrease their activity; a fall in serum calcium results from the decreased rate of bone resorption.

- Calcitonin secretion is stimulated by an increase in serum calcium, and may play a role in preventing postprandial hypercalcemia.

- Calcitonin's role in calcium metabolism is small, however, because persons who have little or no calcitonin following thyroidectomy do not have significant abnormalities in serum calcium levels.

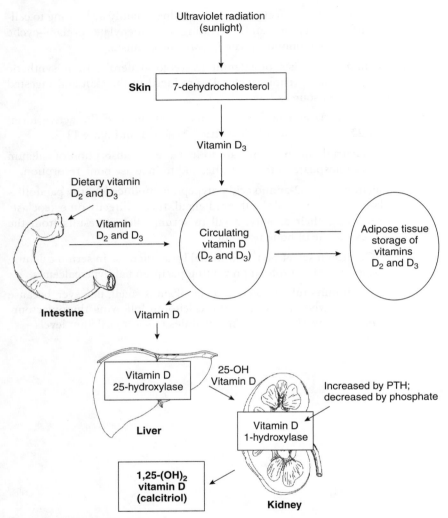

Figure 11-2. Vitamin D metabolism. Ergocalciferol (D$_2$) and cholecalciferol (D$_3$) are converted in the liver to 25-(OH)-cholecalciferol [25-(OH) vitamin D], which in turn is converted to the active form of vitamin D, 1,25-(OH)$_2$ cholecalciferol [1,25-(OH)$_2$ vitamin D, calcitriol] in the kidney. Blood levels of 25-(OH) vitamin D reflect the nutritional supply of Vitamin D, but levels of 1,25-(OH)$_2$ vitamin D are kept relatively constant by the close regulation of the rate of 1-hydroxylation in the kidneys by the blood levels of PTH and phosphate.

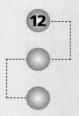

12 Primary Hyperparathyroidism and Other Causes of Hypercalcemia

Increased parathyroid hormone (PTH) production by the parathyroid glands in response to low serum calcium levels is called secondary hyperparathyroidism, and is an appropriate response that tends to return calcium levels toward normal. However, *primary* overproduction of PTH by the parathyroid glands causes a syndrome marked by hypercalcemia and its complications. Hypercalcemia may be caused by other conditions, but in these cases PTH levels are decreased, rather than increased, by the negative feedback effects of the hypercalcemia.

CAUSES AND MANIFESTATIONS OF PRIMARY HYPERPARATHYROIDISM

A single adenoma of one of the parathyroid glands causes 80% to 90% of cases of primary hyperparathyroidism. Hyperplasia of the four glands causes 10% to 20% of cases. Parathyroid carcinoma is a rare cause.

- Increased PTH production by the parathyroid glands leads to hypercalcemia. The manifestations of primary hyperparathyroidism are related mainly to the hypercalcemia and to the effects of PTH on bone and kidneys (Table 12-1).

- Before serum calcium was measured routinely in multichannel chemical analyzers, primary hyperparathyroidism was usually diagnosed in patients with marked hypercalcemia and severe skeletal, renal, and other complications. Now that serum calcium can be measured in routine screening procedures, the disease has been diagnosed more frequently and typically consists of mild hypercalcemia without other manifestations.

Table 12-1. Clinical Manifestations of Primary Hyperparathyroidism
Renal
Urinary calculi
Nephrocalcinosis
Renal failure
Skeletal (osteitis fibrosa cystica)
Demineralization, subperiosteal bone resorption
Bone cysts, "brown tumors"
Neuromuscular
Abnormal mentation
Muscle weakness, fatigue
Gastrointestinal
Anorexia, nausea and vomiting, abdominal pain
Peptic ulcer disease
Pancreatitis

DIAGNOSIS OF PRIMARY HYPERPARATHYROIDISM

 The key to the diagnosis of primary hyperparathyroidism is the finding of elevated serum PTH levels in a patient with hypercalcemia, which is the usual presenting abnormality.

■ Radioimmunoassay of the intact PTH molecule is the preferred diagnostic test, because N-terminal, C-terminal, and mid-molecule fragments are formed during metabolic breakdown of secreted PTH, and assays for these fragments are less representative of the total secretion of the active molecule.

• In addition to hypercalcemia, patients with primary hyperparathyroidism frequently have hypophosphatemia owing to PTH-induced phosphaturia.

• Urine calcium is usually elevated because the hypercalcemia leads to increased glomerular filtration of calcium; however, the increased calcium reabsorption caused by PTH may predominate and prevent hypercalciuria.

■ Benign familial hypercalcemia (familial hypocalciuric hypercalcemia) may be difficult to distinguish from primary hyperparathyroidism. Differentiation from primary hyperparathyroidism depends on the recognition of the familial nature of the disease and the presence of hypocalciuria.

- A genetic defect in the calcium-sensing receptors on the surface of the PTH-producing cells and renal tubular cells leads to an increase in the set-point for serum ionized calcium, and increased renal reabsorption of filtered calcium.

- Persons with benign familial hypercalcemia have slightly-to-moderately increased serum calcium levels, with normal or slightly elevated serum PTH, but *low* urine calcium excretion, which may help explain the lack of renal or skeletal manifestations of the disease.

- Treatment is not necessary. If parathyroidectomy is performed because of failure to recognize the syndrome, the hypercalcemia may not be corrected.

TREATMENT OF PRIMARY HYPERPARATHYROIDISM

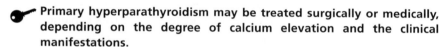 **Primary hyperparathyroidism may be treated surgically or medically, depending on the degree of calcium elevation and the clinical manifestations.**

- ■ The typical patient with primary hyperparathyroidism is an older person who has mild hypercalcemia without complications. This patient may be managed without surgical intervention.

  - If any of the factors listed in Table 12-2 is present, or develops during follow up, surgery is indicated.

Table 12-2. Indications for Surgery in Primary Hyperparathyroidism
Presence of symptoms related to the hypercalcemia
Serum calcium levels greater than 11.4–12.0 mg/dL
Age less than 50 years
Renal manifestations: renal calculi, reduced creatinine clearance, 24-hour urine calcium excretion greater than 400 mg
Bone mineral density more than 2 standard deviations below that of normal persons matched for age, sex, and race
Patient preference for surgery, or unwillingness or inability to undergo prolonged follow up

- Patients whose primary hyperparathyroidism is managed without surgery should be cautioned to avoid dehydration, which might cause sudden renal retention of calcium and increased hypercalcemia.
- Estrogen replacement therapy should be strongly considered for postmenopausal women, who constitute two thirds of the patients with primary hyperparathyroidism, because estrogen tends to lower serum calcium through its effect in decreasing bone resorption.

■ Surgical treatment of primary hyperparathyroidism consists of exploration of the neck and removal of the parathyroid adenoma.

- If parathyroid hyperplasia is found, most or all parathyroid tissue is removed, often with implantation of parathyroid fragments in a location, such as the forearm or neck, that would be convenient if removal of parathyroid tissue is necessary later.
- Ultrasound of the neck and radionuclide parathyroid scans may aid in preoperative tumor localization, but computed tomographic (CT) scans, magnetic resonance imaging (MRI), and venous catheterization studies are usually reserved for cases in which repeat surgery is necessary after unsuccessful neck exploration.

■ After removal of a parathyroid adenoma, the patient may experience a period of hypocalcemia because the remaining normal parathyroid glands have been suppressed by the feedback effects of the prolonged hypercalcemia.

- Occasionally, a patient with severe parathyroid bone disease may have marked hypocalcemia that persists for several months, while serum calcium is taken up by the rapidly remineralizing skeleton (the "hungry bones" syndrome).

HYPERCALCEMIA OF MALIGNANCY

Hypercalcemia may be caused by malignancy, whether bone metastases are present or not.

■ Malignant tumors with bone metastases, such as breast cancer, myeloma, or lymphoma, may cause hypercalcemia by increasing bone resorption. This is caused by local effects, sometimes through the production of locally acting mediators such as osteoclast-activating factor.

■ Malignant tumors may also produce hypercalcemia in the absence of bone metastases. Tumors such as hypernephroma, pancreatic cancer, squamous cell carcinoma of the lung, cervix, or esophagus, and head and neck cancer may produce PTH-related peptide (PTHrP). PTHrP is a humoral factor that binds to PTH receptors and has biologic actions similar to those of PTH, but is not measured in the radio-immunoassay for PTH.

■ Hypercalcemia of malignancy is differentiated from primary hyper-parathyroidism by the finding of an elevated level of PTHrP and a normal or low level of PTH.

OTHER CAUSES OF HYPERCALCEMIA

Hypercalcemia also may be caused by sarcoidosis, hypervitaminosis D, hyperthyroidism, milk-alkali syndrome, thiazide diuretic intake, and Paget's disease.

■ Sarcoidosis sometimes causes hypercalcemia because granulomatous tissue may produce $1,25\text{-}(OH)_2$ vitamin D (calcitriol), leading to increased calcium absorption from the intestine. Activated lymphocytes in the granulomas of sarcoidosis, and other granulomatous diseases such as tuberculosis, histoplasmosis, and leprosy, contain the enzyme vitamin D 1-hydroxylase that converts 25-OH-vitamin D to calcitriol.

■ Hypervitaminosis D most commonly occurs in patients receiving pharmacologic doses of calciferol or calcitriol for the treatment of hypoparathyroidism or chronic renal failure. If the hypercalcemia does not resolve promptly when vitamin D intake is decreased or stopped, glucocorticoids may be used to antagonize the action of vitamin D in the intestine and rapidly decrease calcium absorption.

■ Less common causes of hypercalcemia include the following.

• Hyperthyroidism: Thyroid hormone, like PTH, increases bone resorption.

• Milk-alkali syndrome: Large amounts of absorbable alkali (such as calcium carbonate) and calcium, as were formerly given to treat peptic ulcer disease, may produce hypercalcemia, alkalosis, and renal damage.

• Thiazide diuretics decrease urinary calcium excretion, and should not be used in patients with hyperparathyroidism.

• Paget's disease of bone increases bone turnover. If the patient is immobilized, decreasing the stimuli for bone formation while rapid bone resorption continues because of the Paget's disease, hypercalcemia may result.

MEDICAL TREATMENT OF HYPERCALCEMIA

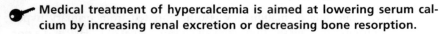 **Medical treatment of hypercalcemia is aimed at lowering serum calcium by increasing renal excretion or decreasing bone resorption.**

- Oral phosphate, in the form of Neutrophos or Fleet Phosphosoda, may be used to lower serum calcium in primary hyperparathyroidism, cancer, and other conditions if definitive therapy is not possible.

  - Extracellular calcification, the main complication of phosphate therapy, is uncommon if no more than 1 to 2 g of phosphate are taken daily.

- In emergency situations, when serum calcium rises higher than 13 to 15 mg/dL and symptoms of hypercalcemia are present, the mainstay of treatment is administration of 4 to 6 L daily of intravenous saline, together with loop diuretics such as furosemide.

  - These measures increase renal calcium excretion by blocking reabsorption of calcium and sodium in the proximal tubules.

- Bisphosphonates lower serum calcium by decreasing bone resorption. Intravenous infusions of pamidronate may be repeated as needed to maintain normal calcium levels.

- Calcitonin blocks the activity of osteoclasts, reducing bone resorption and lowering serum calcium.

  - Calcitonin may be given with a bisphosphonate to combine the earlier onset of action of calcitonin with the longer duration of action of the bisphosphonate.

- Other drugs sometimes useful in the treatment of severe symptomatic hypercalcemia, especially that associated with malignancy, are plicamicin and gallium nitrate.

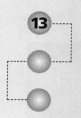

Primary Hypoparathyroidism and Other Causes of Hypocalcemia

Absence of normal parathyroid hormone (PTH) production by the parathyroid glands produces a syndrome marked by hypocalcemia and clinical manifestations related to increased neuromuscular irritability. Hypocalcemia also may be caused by diminished intestinal absorption of calcium due to inadequate availability of dietary calcium or vitamin D, abnormal metabolism or action of vitamin D, or intestinal malabsorption.

CAUSES AND MANIFESTATIONS OF PRIMARY HYPOPARATHYROIDISM

- The most common cause of primary hypoparathyroidism is surgical removal of, or damage to, the parathyroid glands during thyroid surgery or radical neck surgery for cancer.
  - Idiopathic hypoparathyroidism, usually related to autoimmune destruction of the parathyroids, is less common.
- Calcium has an important role in the control of nerve transmission; hypocalcemia causes signs and symptoms related to increased neuromuscular irritability (Table 13-1).

Table 13-1. Manifestations of Primary Hypoparathyroidism

Latent tetany

Muscle fatigue, weakness

Numbness and tingling of hands, feet, mouth

Positive Chvostek's sign* and Trousseau's sign†

Overt tetany

Muscle twitching and cramps

Carpopedal spasm

Laryngeal stridor

Seizures

Long-term effects

Ectodermal changes in nails (atrophy, brittleness, ridging), skin (dryness and scaling), and teeth (enamel defects, hypoplasia)

Calcification of basal ganglia

Cataracts

*Contraction of facial muscles and upper lip after tapping the facial nerve in front of the ear. Present in 10% of normal persons.
†Carpal spasm occurring when a blood pressure cuff on the arm is inflated above systolic pressure for 3 minutes. (Flexion of metacarpophalangeal joints and extension of interphalangeal joints, with flexion of thumb.)

DIAGNOSIS OF PRIMARY HYPOPARATHYROIDISM

 The diagnosis of primary hypoparathyroidism is based on the findings of hypocalcemia and hyperphosphatemia, with low serum PTH levels.

- In addition to the hypocalcemia seen in primary hypoparathyroidism, serum phosphate levels are elevated because of increased renal tubular reabsorption of phosphate in the absence of PTH.

- Urine calcium is decreased because the hypocalcemia leads to diminished glomerular filtration of calcium.

- Pseudohypoparathyroidism is a familial syndrome in which hypocalcemia and hyperphosphatemia are caused by failure of the tissues to respond to PTH, whose levels are normal or elevated.

  - The syndrome of pseudohypoparathyroidism also consists of a group of developmental abnormalities (Albright's hereditary osteodystrophy): short stature, shortening of the metacarpal and metatarsal bones, mental retardation, and other changes.

- Differentiation from primary hypoparathyroidism depends on the presence of the developmental abnormalities, the high rather than low PTH level, and clinical circumstances (i.e., no history of neck surgery, possible family history).

TREATMENT OF PRIMARY HYPOPARATHYROIDISM

Administration of supplemental calcium, with vitamin D to increase its intestinal absorption, will correct the hypocalcemia and hyper-phosphatemia, even when caused by the end-organ unresponsive-ness to PTH of pseudohypoparathyroidism.

- The usual recommended daily intake of calcium in healthy persons is about 1000 mg; persons with primary hypoparathyroidism need an additional 1000 to 2000 mg.
  - Calcium may be given as calcium carbonate, calcium citrate, calcium gluconate, or in other forms.
- Vitamin D is usually given as the active form, calcitriol ($1,25\text{-}(OH)_2$ vitamin D_3, Rocaltrol).
  - Calciferol (ergocalciferol, vitamin D_2) is cheaper, but its onset and cessation of action are slow and unpredictable.
  - Large doses of calciferol must be given, typically 50,000 to 100,000 units daily (compared with a minimum daily requirement of 400 units in healthy persons), because of decreased conversion of ergocalciferol to $1,25\text{-}(OH)_2$ vitamin D in the absence of PTH.

OTHER CAUSES OF HYPOCALCEMIA

- Because nearly half the circulating calcium is bound to protein, hypoalbuminemia causes a decrease in total serum calcium. This is not true hypocalcemia, however, because ionized calcium, which is the biologically active fraction, remains normal. Total serum calcium falls about 0.8 mg/dL for each fall in serum albumin of 1.0 g/dL.
- In persons with chronic renal failure, serum calcium falls because of phosphate retention due to the loss of functioning renal tissue, because of decreased renal production of $1,25\text{-}(OH)_2$ vitamin D, and because of resistance of bone to the action of PTH.
- Hypocalcemia also may be caused by intestinal malabsorption of calcium or vitamin D, or deficiency of vitamin D.

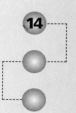

Metabolic Bone Disease

Bone is a living tissue that provides support and protection for body organs, and is active metabolically in the storage and regulation of circulating levels of calcium and phosphorus. Abnormalities in the availability or metabolism of these minerals, or in the function of calciotropic hormones like parathyroid hormone (PTH), calcitonin, and vitamin D, can cause diseases characterized by bone deformity or fractures.

BONE ANATOMY AND PHYSIOLOGY

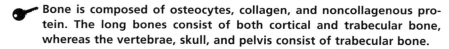 **Bone is composed of osteocytes, collagen, and noncollagenous protein. The long bones consist of both cortical and trabecular bone, whereas the vertebrae, skull, and pelvis consist of trabecular bone.**

- Bone consists of osteocytes embedded in an organic matrix of collagen fibers and noncollagenous protein.

  - The matrix is calcified by the binding of calcium phosphate in the form of hydroxyapatite crystals.

  - Bone is being renewed constantly by a process in which osteoclasts are activated and create resorption cavities, which are then filled in by osteoblasts, replacing old bone with newly formed bone (Fig. 14-1).

    Factors affecting bone resorption and formation are shown in Figure 11-1.

- Cortical (compact) bone is the dense bone that encloses the medullary cavity in the long bones of the extremities.

- Trabecular (cancellous, spongy) bone is composed of a network of thin sheets, or trabeculae. It is found in the ends of the long bones and in the vertebrae, skull, and pelvis.

  - Long bones grow by endochondral ossification: a cartilagenous growth plate between the epiphysis and metaphysis produces a cartilagenous matrix that is eventually replaced by bone.

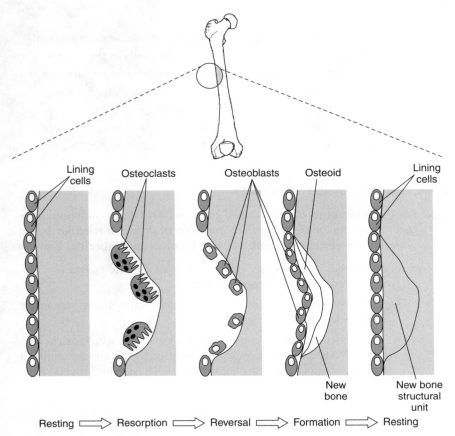

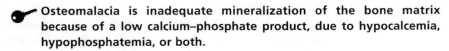

Figure 14-1. Sequence of events in a bone remodeling unit.

OSTEOMALACIA

Osteomalacia is inadequate mineralization of the bone matrix because of a low calcium–phosphate product, due to hypocalcemia, hypophosphatemia, or both.

- The classic cause is vitamin D deficiency, but osteomalacia also may be caused by abnormalities of vitamin D metabolism, renal phosphate loss, or failure of intestinal absorption of calcium, phosphate, or vitamin D.

■ Rickets is a severe form of osteomalacia that occurs in children before closure of the cartilagenous growth plates. Bowing of the long bones and widening of the epiphyses occur, with bone pain and tenderness and muscle weakness.

■ Treatment of osteomalacia consists of providing adequate amounts of vitamin D and calcium.

• Less often, correction of a reversible abnormality such as malabsorption is needed.

OSTEOPOROSIS

Osteoporosis is a decrease in the total amount of bone, along with defects in microarchitecture such as thinning and loss of connecting and supporting trabeculae. The bone that remains is histologically normal, but the loss of bone mass and compromise of architectural integrity increases the susceptibility to fractures.

■ Bone mass reaches a peak by age 30, and then declines by about 1% per year.

• A more rapid decline (2% to 3% per year) occurs in women in the years immediately after menopause, because of estrogen deficiency.

• Bone mineral density, as measured by dual energy absorptiometry (DEXA), that is more than 1 standard deviation (SD) below estimated peak bone density indicates *osteopenia*; more than 2.5 SD indicates *osteoporosis*.

■ There are several causes of osteoporosis. Specific risk factors for osteoporosis in women are listed in Table 14-1.

• Low bone mass at maturity, which is partly related to genetic and ethnic factors, is one cause.

Table 14-1. Risk Factors for Osteoporosis in Women
Caucasian (especially northern European) or Asian ancestry
Short stature, slender build, small bones
Family history of osteoporosis
Smoking history, excess alcohol intake
Estrogen deficiency: early menopause; normal menopause without estrogen replacement

- Deficiency of sex steroids, as occurs in postmenopausal women and in men with hypogonadism, can result in osteoporosis.

- Calcium deficiency can lead to increased bone resorption by PTH to maintain serum calcium levels, causing osteoporosis.

- Secondary osteoporosis may occur with glucocorticoid therapy, Cushing's syndrome, malabsorption of calcium or vitamin D, myeloma, or prolonged immobilization.

■ Clinical manifestations of osteoporosis are related to the increased risk of fractures, especially of the spine, hips, and wrists.

- Wedge fractures or compression fractures of the thoracic vertebrae may lead to loss of height and dorsal kyphosis.

- Hip fractures are followed by permanent disability in 50% of cases, and death due to complications such as pulmonary embolism or pneumonia occurs in 10% to 20% of the elderly persons who suffer these fractures.

Osteoporosis may be treated with calcium and vitamin D supplementation, estrogen replacement (in postmenopausal women), and other antiresorptive agents (which include, in addition to estrogen bisphospaonates and calcitonin.) (Fig. 14-2).

■ Patients with osteoporosis should consume at least 1500 mg of calcium daily, which often requires calcium supplements of 1000 mg.

- Vitamin D intake of 400 to 800 units daily should be assured, with supplements if needed.

■ Estrogen replacement therapy after menopause decreases the bone-resorbing action of PTH, leading to increased bone density and decreased fracture rate.

- Because it has other potential benefits, estrogen replacement is the first treatment to consider (in addition to calcium and vitamin D supplementation) in postmenopausal women.

■ Bisphosphonates (e.g., alendronate and risedronate) bind to the hydroxyapatite crystals in bone and, when ingested by osteoclasts, inhibit the action of the osteoclasts in producing bone resorption. Their effect in increasing bone density and decreasing the fracture rate is similar to that of estrogen.

■ Calcitonin, given by injection or by nasal spray, inhibits the action of osteoclasts and increases bone density; however, its beneficial effect

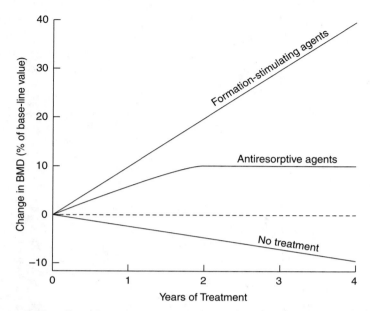

Figure 14-2. The effect of antiresorptive and formation-stimulating agents on bone mineral density in osteoporosis. Because resorption cavities make up about 10% of bone volume, agents that stop resorption while allowing formation to continue may produce up to a 10% increase in bone density as the cavities fill in with new bone over 6 to 24 months; further increase may not occur, but the expected gradual decrease in bone density is prevented. Formation-stimulating agents, in contrast, could lead to continuing increase in bone density.

on fracture rate is less well established than that of estrogen and bisphosphonates.

■ Agents that stimulate bone formation include fluoride and low doses of PTH. These are still investigational agents for the treatment of osteoporosis, however.

Glucose Metabolism and Diabetes Mellitus

15 Insulin and Glucose Homeostasis

Blood glucose levels and utilization of glucose for energy production or glycogen storage are closely regulated by feedback-controlled secretion of insulin and glucagon.

INSULIN AND THE ISLETS OF LANGERHANS

The islets of Langerhans are groups of endocrine cells, with approximately 1000 cells in each islet, scattered throughout the parenchymal tissue of the pancreas. Four cell types are recognized: alpha cells produce glucagon; beta cells produce insulin; delta cells produce somatostatin; and PP cells produce pancreatic polypeptide.

■ Insulin is a 51-amino acid protein consisting of an A chain and a B chain linked by two sulfhydryl groups (Fig. 15-1). Its parent molecule, proinsulin, splits to release insulin and equimolar amounts of connecting peptide (C-peptide).

• Insulin acts by binding to the extracellular portion of its specific membrane receptor, which leads to autophosphorylation of the intracellular portion of the receptor at its tyrosine residues. This stimulates tyrosine protein kinase activity, leading to intracellular effects that mediate insulin's action.

For example, in muscle and fat cells the activity of a glucose transporter (GLUT-4) is stimulated, increasing the transport of glucose across the cell membrane and into the cells.

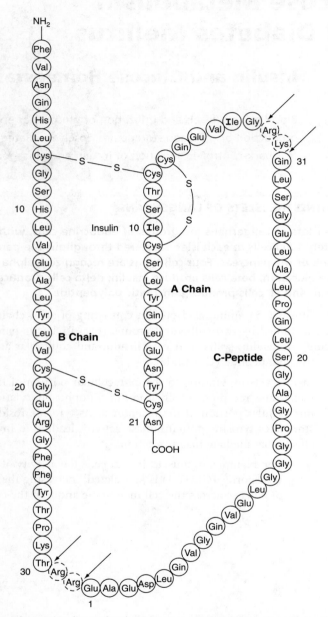

Figure 15-1. The proinsulin molecule. Cleavage at the sites indicated by the *arrows* removes C-peptide and four amino acid residues, leaving the insulin molecule. (Adapted from Murray RK, et al: *Harper's Biochemistry,* 23rd ed. Stanford, CT, Appleton & Lange, 1993, p 560.)

GLUCOSE HOMEOSTASIS

 Glucose and insulin function in a negative-feedback loop to maintain normal levels of serum glucose.

- Glucose is the main stimulus for insulin secretion by the pancreatic beta cell.

  - A membrane glucose transporter (GLUT-2) carries glucose from the bloodstream into the beta cell, where it is phosphorylated by glucokinase, and undergoes glycolysis and oxidation to carbon dioxide and water. This process recruits calcium ions, which cause granules containing proinsulin to move to the cell surface, undergo exocytosis, and release insulin and C-peptide into the circulation.

  - The secretion of insulin induced by glucose constitutes a negative-feedback loop that maintains serum glucose levels in a narrow range of about 70 to 90 mg/dL in the fasting state, and prevents glucose levels from rising much above 125 mg/dL after a meal.

- The liver also helps maintain normal glucose levels.

  - When glucose floods into the bloodstream from the gastrointestinal tract following a meal, glucose disposal is aided by hepatic formation and storage of glycogen. During periods of fasting, the liver helps prevent a decrease in blood glucose by releasing glucose from glycogen stores (glycogenolysis) and by producing glucose through gluconeogenesis.

- Insulin's main effects on glucose homeostasis are the stimulation of glucose utilization by peripheral tissues and the suppression of hepatic glucose output. Insulin promotes the storage of glucose as glycogen, amino acids as protein, and fatty acids as triglycerides.

  - Insulin stimulates the transfer of glucose across the cell membrane and into the cytoplasm of liver, muscle, and fat cells, and it promotes glycogen formation by stimulating glucose phosphorylation and glycogen synthase activity in liver and muscle cells.

  - Insulin promotes fat storage through its antilipolytic action, which decreases free fatty acid and triglyceride release from fat.

  - Insulin has anabolic and anticatabolic effects in muscle, decreasing protein breakdown and enhancing amino acid uptake and protein formation.

- Glucagon acts as a counterregulatory hormone to insulin. Its release is prompted by a fall in blood glucose, which it counteracts by increasing hepatic glucose output through stimulation of glycogenolysis and gluconeogenesis.

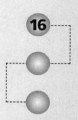

16 Pathogenesis and Diagnosis of Diabetes Mellitus

Diabetes mellitus is a disorder of glucose metabolism in which the action of insulin on body cells is inadequate, either because of impaired insulin production or because of a combination of impaired insulin production and resistance of target tissues to insulin's actions.

PATHOGENESIS OF DIABETES MELLITUS

About 10% of patients with diabetes have type 1 diabetes, formerly called *insulin-dependent diabetes mellitus (IDDM)*; 90% have type 2 diabetes, formerly called *non–insulin-dependent diabetes mellitus (NIDDM)*. The main differences between the two types of diabetes are shown in Table 16-1.

- In type 1 diabetes, insulin production is virtually absent because of beta-cell destruction. The causes of this destruction include genetic

Table 16-1. Characteristics of Type 1 and Type 2 Diabetes Mellitus

	Type 1 Diabetes Mellitus	Type 2 Diabetes Mellitus
Prevalence	0.2%–0.5%; men = women	4%–6%; women > men
Age at onset	Usually < 25 years	Usually > 40 years
Genetics	<10% of first-degree relatives affected; 50% concordance in identical twins	>20% of first-degree relatives affected; 90%–100% concordance in identical twins
HLA	Associated with HLA-DR3, HLA-DR4, HLA-DQ	None
Autoimmunity	Increased prevalence of autoantibodies to islet cells and other tissues	None
Body build	Usually lean	Usually obese
Metabolism	Ketosis prone; insulin production absent	Ketosis resistant; insulin levels may be high, normal, or low
Treatment	Insulin	Weight loss; oral agents and insulin if needed

factors, autoimmunity, and perhaps environmental factors (e.g., viral infection coincident with the initial diagnosis of diabetes).

- Antibodies to islet-cell antigens, especially glutamic acid decarboxylase (anti-GAD) are commonly present for many years before, and sometimes for several years after, the onset of clinical diabetes.

- The onset of clinical diabetes occurs when progressive destruction of the beta cells has left too little residual insulin production to maintain glucose tolerance.

■ In type 2 diabetes, insulin production is impaired but not totally absent; in addition, insulin resistance, most commonly associated with obesity, is present.

- Obese persons whose insulin production can increase enough to compensate for the insulin resistance maintain normal glucose tolerance; presumably, the combination of obesity-associated insulin resistance with beta-cell impairment results in type 2 diabetes.

■ The main clinical difference between type 1 and type 2 diabetes is that the total absence of insulin in type 1 disease results in ketoacidosis unless treatment is given; thus, the description "insulin dependent." Patients with type 2 disease also may require insulin for optimal glucose control, but the persistence of some insulin activity prevents the development of ketoacidosis.

DIAGNOSIS OF DIABETES MELLITUS

■ Diabetes mellitus is diagnosed if any of the following abnormalities is present on two occasions.

- Fasting plasma glucose level of 126 mg/dL or greater

- Plasma glucose level of 200 mg/dL or greater 2 hours after a 75-g glucose load (i.e., oral glucose tolerance test)

- Casual or random plasma glucose level (i.e., without regard to food intake) of 200 mg/dL or greater, with symptoms of diabetes

■ The category "impaired fasting glucose" or "impaired glucose tolerance" recognizes a stage between normal glucose tolerance and overt diabetes in which symptomatic hyperglycemia may be absent, but there is increased risk for the atherosclerotic complications of diabetes, and for the development of overt diabetes in the future.

- Impaired fasting glucose is present if the fasting plasma glucose level is greater than 110 mg/dL but less than 126 mg/dL.

- Impaired glucose tolerance is present if the plasma glucose level is 140 mg/dL or greater, but less than 200 mg/dL, 2 hours after a 75-gram glucose load.

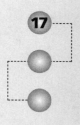

Manifestations and Acute Complications of Diabetes

The manifestations of diabetes mellitus include symptoms caused directly by the hyperglycemia; acute metabolic complications, diabetic ketoacidosis and hyperosmolar nonketotic coma; and long-term complications.

SYMPTOMS OF HYPERGLYCEMIA

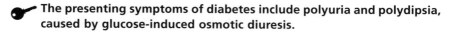 **The presenting symptoms of diabetes include polyuria and polydipsia, caused by glucose-induced osmotic diuresis.**

■ Weight loss and weakness, despite increased food intake, result from the urinary glucose loss and from lack of the anabolic effects of insulin.

■ Infections of the skin, vulva, urinary tract, and elsewhere are related to hyperglycemia-induced loss of resistance to infection.

■ Osmotic changes in the optic lens alter its shape and refractive qualities, causing blurred vision.

DIABETIC KETOACIDOSIS

In untreated type 1 diabetes, the insulin deficit is severe enough to shift hepatic fuel production toward ketogenesis. Loss of the antilipolytic action of insulin increases the release from fat cells of free fatty acids, which are taken up by the liver. Glucagon, unopposed by insulin, increases hepatic levels of carnitine, enabling fatty acids to enter the mitochondria and undergo beta-oxidation to acetoacetate and beta-hydroxybutyrate. Glucagon also decreases hepatic malonyl coenzyme A, an inhibitor of fatty acid oxidation. The series of events shown in Figure 17-1 leads to diabetic ketoacidosis.

■ Diabetic ketoacidosis is suggested by rapid worsening of glycemic control, often precipitated by omission of insulin doses or acute stress due to illness or injury.

• Patients may have altered mental status, gastrointestinal symptoms such as vomiting or abdominal pain, and physical findings of dehydration, hypotension, and rapid deep breathing (Kussmaul's respiration) due to the acidosis.

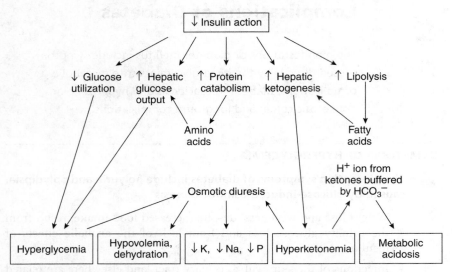

Figure 17-1. Pathogenesis of diabetic ketoacidosis. Decreased insulin action affects many organs and metabolic processes, leading to the manifestations of diabetic ketoacidosis shown in the bottom row of the diagram.

- Laboratory findings include a serum glucose level greater than 250 mg/dL, a positive test for serum and urine ketones, and evidence of acidosis (i.e., serum bicarbonate lower than 10 mEq/L, serum pH lower than 7.25). Serum levels of sodium, potassium, and phosphorus are low, although potassium levels may be elevated initially because of potassium ion movement from the intracellular to the extracellular space.

TREATMENT OF DIABETIC KETOACIDOSIS

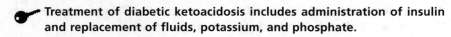 **Treatment of diabetic ketoacidosis includes administration of insulin and replacement of fluids, potassium, and phosphate.**

- ■ Insulin is given to increase tissue utilization of glucose, to inhibit the flow of fatty acids and amino acids from peripheral tissues, and to reverse the hepatic production of ketones.

  - Initial doses of 5 to 10 units per hour intravenously will provide maximal insulin effect; the rate of infusion is decreased as the hyperglycemia and ketoacidosis are corrected.

- ■ Fluid replacement with saline solution is needed to correct the dehydration and hypovolemia; the average deficit is 3 to 5 L.

  - • Glucose solutions are infused when serum glucose has fallen to 200 to 300 mg/dL, to prevent hypoglycemia.

- ■ Potassium must be replaced with potassium choloride or potassium phosphate; however, this is delayed until serum potassium levels, which may be elevated initially, have become normal or low.

- ■ Phosphate must also be replaced. Bicarbonate is given only when the acidosis is very severe, with pH below 6.9 to 7.1.

HYPERGLYCEMIC HYPEROSMOLAR NONKETOTIC COMA

🔑 **Hyperglycemic hyperosmolar nonketotic coma is a complication that typically occurs in type 2 rather than type 1 diabetes. Because insulin levels are high enough to prevent ketoacidosis, the manifestations are related mainly to the marked glucose elevations (>600 mg/dL) and resulting hyperosmolality (>320 mOsm/kg) and osmotic diuresis that lead to dehydration and altered mental status.**

- ■ The cause of the severe hyperglycemia may be an intercurrent illness or other stress in an elderly diabetic patient whose fluid intake does not keep pace with the glucose-induced water loss; the resulting dehydration impairs renal function, decreasing urinary glucose output and thus further increasing the hyperglycemia.

- ■ Treatment of hyperglycemic hyperosmolar nonketotic coma is similar to the treatment of diabetic ketoacidosis, except that fluid replacement is the first priority because the severe hypovolemia may lead to shock or thromboembolism.

  - • Fluid replacement may lower glucose levels, independent of the action of insulin, through its effect in improving renal function.

  - • Insulin therapy should not be started until fluid replacement is underway: the hyperglycemia actually may help to maintain extracellular volume, and lowering glucose levels before correcting the hypovolemia may increase the risk of shock.

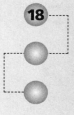

Chronic Complications of Diabetes

The long-term morbidity associated with diabetes is caused by microvascular changes that affect the eyes and kidneys; by changes in the peripheral and autonomic nervous system; and by macrovascular changes (atherosclerosis) that affect the medium and large arteries.

PATHOGENESIS OF CHRONIC COMPLICATIONS

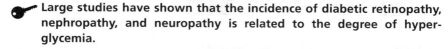 **Large studies have shown that the incidence of diabetic retinopathy, nephropathy, and neuropathy is related to the degree of hyperglycemia.**

- More intensive treatment that led to more effective glycemic control has decreased the incidence of complications in type 1 diabetes (Diabetes Control and Complications Trial)[1] and type 2 diabetes (United Kingdom Prospective Diabetes Study).[2]

- It is not known how hyperglycemia causes damage to small and large blood vessels and other tissues. Possible mechanisms include the nonenzymatic glycosylation of proteins (which is similar to the process that produces glycosylated hemoglobin) and tissue damage related to the conversion of glucose to sorbitol by the enzyme aldose reductase.

DIABETIC RETINOPATHY

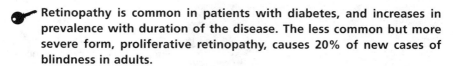 **Retinopathy is common in patients with diabetes, and increases in prevalence with duration of the disease. The less common but more severe form, proliferative retinopathy, causes 20% of new cases of blindness in adults.**

- Background (simple, nonproliferative) retinopathy makes up 90% to 95% of cases of retinopathy. It consists of venous dilatation, exudates, hemorrhages, and microaneurysms on funduscopic examination (Fig. 18-1B).

---

[1] The Diabetes Control and Complications Trial Research Group. The effect of intensive treatment of diabetes on the development and progression of long-term complications in insulin-dependent diabetes mellitus. N. Engl J. Med. 1993;329:977–86.

[2] UK Prospective Diabetes Study (UKPDS) Group. Intensive blood-glucose control with sulphonylureas or insulin compared with conventional treatment and risk of complications in patients with type 2 diabetes (UKPDS 83). Lancet. 1998;352:837.

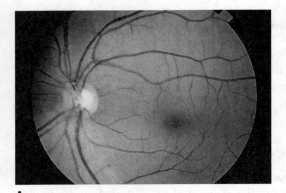

A

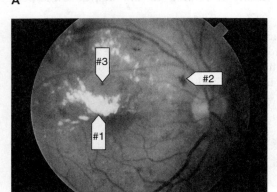

B

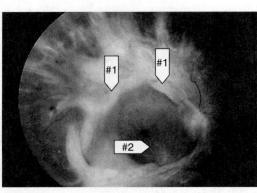

C

Figure 18-1. Diabetic retinopathy. (*A*) Normal retina. (*B*) Background diabetic retinopathy, with hard exudates (*arrow 1*), hemorrhages (*arrow 2*), and microaneurysms (*arrow 3*). (*C*) Proliferative retinopathy, with glial proliferation (*arrow 1*) causing tractional retinal detachment (*arrow 2*). (Courtesy of Stephen W. Wong, M.D.)

- These changes are caused by increased capillary permeability, vascular occlusion, and weakness of supporting structures.

■ Proliferative retinopathy, which makes up 5% to 10% of cases, threatens vision.

- Vascular occlusion and ischemia cause neovascularization. New vessels form on the retinal surface, and preretinal or vitreous hemorrhage may lead to scarring and retinal detachment (Fig. 18-1C).

■ Annual screening of diabetic patients for retinopathy may allow earlier treatment and prevent blindness.

- Laser-beam photocoagulation may obliterate new vessels, and vitrectomy may improve vision in patients with vitreous hemorrhage and scarring.

DIABETIC NEPHROPATHY

🔑 Significant renal disease occurs in about 40% of patients with type 1 diabetes and 20% of patients with type 2 diabetes.

■ The most characteristic renal lesion is intercapillary glomerulosclerosis, characterized by deposits in the mesangial matrix, widening of the glomerular basement membrane, and hyalinization of the afferent and efferent arterioles (Fig. 18-2).

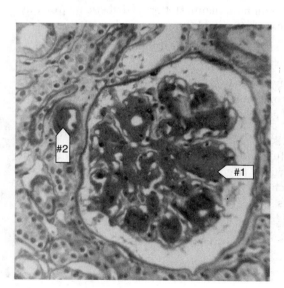

Figure 18-2. Diabetic nephropathy, with nodular intercapillary glomerulosclerosis (original magnification × 160). The mesangium is diffusely increased, with one large mesangial nodule (*arrow 1*) and several smaller nodules. Hyaline deposits are present in an arteriole (*arrow 2*). (Courtesy of I. Bruce Elfenbein, M.D.)

■ Microalbuminuria (excretion of 30 to 300 mg albumin in 24 hours) may be the earliest sign of diabetic nephropathy. This may progress to proteinuria (excretion of more than 300 mg in 24 hours), then to the nephrotic syndrome and end-stage renal disease.

- Almost one third of new cases of end-stage renal disease are caused by diabetes.

- Coexisting hypertension is associated with a marked increase in the risk of rapid progression of renal disease.

■ Measures that may slow the progression of renal disease are intensive blood glucose management, control of hypertension, and limitation of dietary protein intake.

- Angiotensin-converting-enzyme inhibitors (e.g., captopril) are especially effective in decreasing proteinuria and the progression of renal failure.

DIABETIC NEUROPATHY

🔑 Neuropathy occurs in at least 50% of patients with long-standing diabetes. Nerve conduction velocity is slowed, and loss of large-diameter nerve fibers occurs.

■ Peripheral neuropathy causing paresthesias and pain in the lower extremities is the most common manifestation of diabetic neuropathy. Weakness and upper extremity involvement occur less often.

- Examination often shows decreased deep-tendon reflexes and loss of pain and vibratory sensation.

■ Autonomic neuropathy also may occur, causing postural hypotension, sexual impotence, urinary retention, and abnormal gastrointestinal motility with delayed gastric emptying, constipation, or diarrhea.

■ Improved glucose control lowers the risk of progressive neuropathy.

- Treatment of painful neuropathy is often unsatisfactory. Tricyclic antidepressant drugs (e.g., amitriptyline, imipramine, and desipramine), which block central pain transmission pathways, are the first-line agents.

ATHEROSCLEROSIS

 Coronary artery disease is twice as common in patients with diabetes, compared with nondiabetic persons.

- The risk of myocardial infarction may be decreased by effective control of glucose levels.

- Peripheral vascular disease affecting the lower extremities in persons with diabetes may lead to ischemia, ulceration, and infection. Disease sometimes progresses to gangrene and the need for amputation is a significant risk.

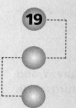

Management of Diabetes

Treatment with diet and exercise, insulin, and oral agents can correct the hyperglycemia and other metabolic abnormalities of diabetes. Treatment that lowers serum glucose levels but does not produce normoglycemia may relieve the symptoms and prevent the acute complications of diabetes, but more intensive treatment will provide greater protection against the long-term complications of the disease.

DIET AND EXERCISE

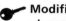 **Modifications in diet and an increase in physical activity can improve glycemic control.**

- Principles of dietary treatment of diabetes include the following.
  - Limit carbohydrate intake, especially rapidly absorbed simple sugars, to minimize hyperglycemia.
  - Limit consumption of saturated fat and cholesterol to protect against the long-term complication of atherosclerosis.
  - Adjust calorie intake to achieve ideal weight. (Limiting calorie intake usually is required.)

    A typical distribution of calorie intake might be 10% to 20% protein, 50% to 60% carbohydrate, and 20% to 30% fat.

  - Maintain regular and appropriate timing of food intake to match the pattern of insulin and oral agent use.
- Regular exercise increases glucose utilization by muscle and fat cells, and can improve glycemic control.
  - An episode of greater-than-usual physical activity may lead to hypoglycemia, unless food intake is increased or insulin dosage is decreased.

ORAL ANTIHYPERGLYCEMIC DRUGS

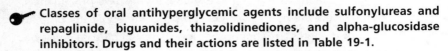 Classes of oral antihyperglycemic agents include sulfonylureas and repaglinide, biguanides, thiazolidinediones, and alpha-glucosidase inhibitors. Drugs and their actions are listed in Table 19-1.

- Sulfonylureas and repaglinide act on the beta cells of the islets of Langerhaus to increase insulin release.

  - These drugs bind to receptors on the beta cells, resulting in the closing of adenosine triphosphate (ATP)-dependent potassium channels and consequent depolarization of the cell membrane. This causes the opening of calcium channels and influx of calcium into the cell, which in turn causes movement of insulin secretory granules to the cell membrane and secretion of insulin.

  - To some extent, this process is dependent on the serum glucose level; that is, these drugs produce greater stimulation of insulin output when hyperglycemia is present (e.g., following a meal).

  - Hypoglycemia is the most significant complication of sulfonylurea therapy.

Table 19-1. Oral Antihyperglycemic Drugs

	Sulfonylureas and repaglinide	Biguanides	Thiazolidinediones	Alpha-glucosidase Inhibitors
Drugs	Glyburide, glipizide, glimepiride, chlorpropamide, tolbutamide, tolazamide, acetohexamide, repaglinide (a benzoic acid derivative)	Metformin	Rosiglitazone, pioglitazone	Acarbose, miglitol
Action	Increase in insulin secretion	Inhibition of hepatic glucose output; increase in insulin sensitivity in peripheral tissues (lesser effect)	Increase in peripheral sensitivity to insulin	Decrease in gastrointestinal absorption of glucose

- Metformin, a biguanide, reduces hepatic glucose output by decreasing hepatic gluconeogenesis and glycogenolysis, and may increase sensitivity to insulin in muscle and other tissues.

  - Because insulin output is not increased, hypoglycemia is not a direct result of metformin use, and the weight gain commonly seen with insulin therapy, and with use of sulfonylureas, does not occur.

  - The limiting factors in the use of metformin often are gastrointestinal side effects such as diarrhea and abdominal discomfort. A low initial dose, with gradual increases, will minimize this problem.

  - Lactic acidosis is a rare, but serious, complication. Metformin should not be given to patients who have renal insufficiency, liver disease, or cardiac or pulmonary conditions that might cause decreased oxygenation of peripheral tissues; most cases of lactic acidosis have occurred in such patients.

- The thiazolidinediones include rosiglitazone and pioglitazone. They act mainly by increasing the sensitivity of muscle and adipose tissue to insulin.

  - The thiazolidinediones bind to the peroxisome proliferator-activated receptor (PPAR) in these tissues, increasing the expression of glucose transporters (GLUT-1, GLUT-4), which mediate insulin's effects on glucose utilization.

  - A lesser action of the thiazolidinediones is the inhibition of hepatic glucose output.

  - Hepatotoxicity, sometimes fatal, has occurred in patients taking thiazolidinediones. Liver disease is a contraindication to the use of thiazolidinediones; liver function tests should be performed regularly in patients taking these drugs.

- Alpha-glucosidase inhibitors (e.g., acarbose and meglitol) are complex oligosaccharides that competitively inhibit the enzymes that hydrolyze polysaccharides to glucose and other monosaccharides in the brush border of the small intestine. This action delays the digestion and absorption of glucose, blunting the increase in blood glucose that occurs after a meal.

  - The antihyperglycemic effect of these drugs is less than that of sulfonylureas, biguanides, or thiazolidinediones, and affects the postprandial glucose levels more than the fasting levels.

■ The main side effects of alpha-glucosidase inhibitors are flatulence, crampy abdominal pain, and diarrhea. Low initial doses and gradual upward titration are necessary to minimize the gastrointestinal side effects.

INSULIN

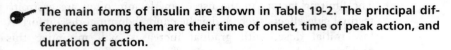 **The main forms of insulin are shown in Table 19-2. The principal differences among them are their time of onset, time of peak action, and duration of action.**

■ The simplest regimen is a single dose of intermediate-acting insulin before breakfast. This will lower glucose levels during the day, but may or may not maintain satisfactory control for 24 hours.

• If the morning glucose level remains elevated with a single morning dose of insulin, a second dose of intermediate-acting insulin may be added before supper or at bedtime.

The morning dose is regulated according to the afternoon glucose level, and the evening dose according to the morning level.

■ Intensive insulin therapy with three or more daily insulin injections or with a portable infusion pump may be chosen if glucose levels are

Table 19-2. Insulin Preparations and Their Onset, Peak, and Approximate Duration of Action

Types	Onset of Action (h)	Peak Effect (h)	Duration of Action (h)
Fast Acting			
Regular human insulin	0.5	2.5–5	8
Insulin lispro	0.25	0.5–1.5	4
Intermediate Acting			
NPH human insulin	1.5	4–12	24
Lente insulin	2.5	7–15	24
70% NPH human, 30% regular human insulin	0.5	2–12	24
Long Acting			
Ultralente insulin	4	10–30	36

unstable, or if the patient accepts the increased inconvenience in order to achieve the best possible glucose control.

■ A dose of fast-acting insulin may be given before each meal to control the postprandial rise in serum glucose, while basal insulin requirements are supplied by a single morning or evening dose of a long-acting insulin.

> Insulin doses in this regimen are adjusted frequently according to fingerstick glucose determinations.

■ The closest possible control of serum glucose can be achieved by the constant subcutaneous infusion of regular insulin by a portable pump. A basal rate of infusion is supplemented by bolus doses before each meal.

> This treatment may be limited by its inconvenience for the patient and by the increased risk of hypoglycemia.

CHOICE OF TREATMENT

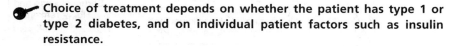 **Choice of treatment depends on whether the patient has type 1 or type 2 diabetes, and on individual patient factors such as insulin resistance.**

■ In persons with type 1 diabetes, insulin must be given to prevent diabetic ketoacidosis and to maintain the best possible glycemic control. Oral antihyperglycemic agents have no role in treatment of type 1 diabetes.

■ In type 2 diabetes, it is desirable to avoid the use of insulin if possible, because insulin may stimulate appetite and promote further weight gain in patients whose glucose intolerance is commonly related to obesity and insulin resistance. Also, the high doses of insulin that are often needed in patients with type 2 diabetes are suspected of being atherogenic.

• Achievement of glycemic control with one or more antihyperglycemic oral agents should be attempted, unless extremely high glucose levels mandate the initial (it is hoped temporary) use of insulin.

• If treatment with oral agents provides unsatisfactory control of plasma glucose levels, a small dose of intermediate-acting insulin can be added at bedtime.

This may inhibit excessive hepatic glucose output during the night, thus lowering the fasting morning glucose level and increasing the ability of oral agents to maintain normal glucose levels through the day.

■ A scheme for the suggested use of oral agents and insulin in patients with type 2 diabetes is shown in Figure 19-1.

  • The measurement of hemoglobin A_{1C} or glycosylated hemoglobin, which reflects the average blood glucose levels during the preceding 6 to 12 weeks, is useful along with fasting glucose measurements in evaluating the adequacy of treatment.

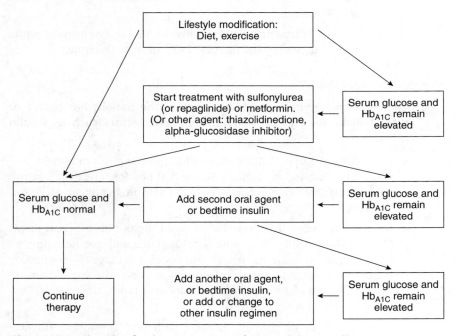

Figure 19-1. Algorithm for the management of type 2 diabetes mellitus.

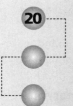

Hypoglycemia

Low blood sugar may be caused by excessive insulin production or administration, or by metabolic abnormalities that affect the liver's ability to maintain glucose levels between meals. An insulin-secreting tumor of the beta cells of the islets of Langerhans is a rare cause, but must be ruled out because of its serious manifestations.

MANIFESTATIONS OF HYPOGLYCEMIA

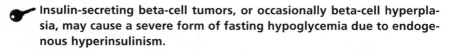 **Hypoglycemia is often defined as a serum glucose level below 45 mg/dL, but the level at which symptoms occur may be higher or lower in different persons and at different times in the same person. Clinical hypoglycemia is better defined by the presence of "Whipple's triad": low serum glucose; the presence of typical hypoglycemic symptoms; and relief of symptoms when the glucose level rises.**

■ The early symptoms of hypoglycemia usually are caused by the increase in catecholamine levels and sympathetic outflow that occur in response to the fall in serum glucose levels.

- These adrenergic symptoms include sweating, tachycardia, palpitations, tremulousness, lightheadedness, and muscle weakness.

- If hypoglycemia is prolonged, glucose deprivation in the central nervous system may produce mental changes that progress from somnolence and confusion to coma, along with headache, slurred speech, focal neurologic changes, and seizures.

INSULINOMA

Insulin-secreting beta-cell tumors, or occasionally beta-cell hyperplasia, may cause a severe form of fasting hypoglycemia due to endogenous hyperinsulinism.

■ A key to the diagnosis of insulinoma is the demonstration that serum insulin levels remain high despite hypoglycemia, because normal beta cells stop producing insulin when serum glucose levels fall.

- For example, if the serum glucose level is less than 45 mg/dL, a serum insulin level greater than 10 mU/ml is abnormal and suggests the presence of an insulinoma.

A prolonged fast, up to 72 hours, may be necessary to induce the hypoglycemia that will make it possible to demonstrate this abnormality.

■ Factitious hypoglycemia also may be accompanied by inappropriately high insulin levels.

• Surreptitious insulin injection must be ruled out by showing detectable C-peptide levels (which normally accompany endogenous insulin secretion but would be suppressed by exogenous insulin).

• Surreptitious sulfonylurea ingestion must be ruled out by screening blood or urine for these drugs.

■ If the diagnosis remains uncertain after a prolonged fast, a C- peptide suppression test may be done.

• In a C-peptide suppression test, a 1-hour intravenous insulin infusion (0.1 unit/kg) is given to induce hypoglycemia.

• C-peptide normally is suppressed by the hypoglycemia; a level that remains high indicates an insulinoma. (C-peptide is measured rather than insulin because the exogenous insulin would make impossible the interpretation of insulin levels.)

■ Insulinomas may be visualized by magnetic resonance imaging (MRI) or computed tomographic (CT) scanning, or by intraoperative ultrasound.

• If surgical removal is not possible, medical treatment with diazoxide can inhibit the release of insulin by beta cells.

OTHER CAUSES OF HYPOGLYCEMIA

■ Postprandial reactive hypoglycemia may occur in gastrectomized patients.

• In these patients, it is caused by rapid movement of food into the small bowel, with rapid carbohydrate absorption stimulating excess insulin production (alimentary hypoglycemia).

■ "Idiopathic" or "functional" reactive hypoglycemia has been over-diagnosed in the past because of misinterpretation of the 5-hour glucose tolerance test. Many normal persons have serum glucose levels of 40 to 55 mg/dL, without hypoglycemic symptoms, after the non-physiologic stimulus of 75 to 100 g of glucose.

- Most patients with hypoglycemia-like symptoms after meals do not have low glucose levels.

- In the occasional true case of functional reactive hypoglycemia (i.e., one that fulfills the criteria of Whipple's triad), treatment consists of multiple small meals that are high in protein and low in carbohydrate.

■ Ethanol-induced hypoglycemia may occur 12 to 24 hours after a period of heavy drinking. Gluconeogenesis may be inhibited because nicotinamide adenine dinucleotide (NAD), needed for gluconeogenesis, is converted to reduced nicotinamide adenine dinucleotide (NADH) when alcohol is oxidized to acetaldehyde and acetate.

- If glycogen stores are depleted because of inadequate recent food intake, the additional insult of decreased ability to perform gluconeogenesis may result in hypoglycemia.

■ Other causes of hypoglycemia include large intra-abdominal tumors, liver disease, kidney disease, and sepsis.

The Adrenal Glands

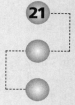

21   Adrenal Anatomy and Physiology

The adrenal cortex produces hormones that affect carbohydrate metabolism, immune function, response to stress, sodium and potassium balance, sexual function, and other processes. These hormones are regulated mainly by pituitary adrenocorticotropic hormone (ACTH) and by the renin–angiotensin system. The adrenal medulla is closely related to the sympathetic nervous system, and produces catecholamines, which contribute to the actions of the sympathetic nervous system.

ADRENAL ANATOMY

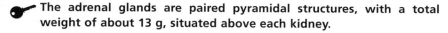 **The adrenal glands are paired pyramidal structures, with a total weight of about 13 g, situated above each kidney.**

■ The adrenal cortex is of mesodermal origin. It is divided into three zones: the outer zone (glomerulosa) produces aldosterone; the middle zone (fasciculata) produces cortisol; and the inner zone (reticularis) produces androgens and estrogens.

■ The adrenal medulla is derived from neural ectoderm. It is composed mainly of chromaffin cells, so named because a colored pigment is formed from oxidation of catecholamines when the cells are stained with potassium dichromate.

   • Chromaffin cells are also present in sympathetic ganglia and elsewhere.

SYNTHESIS OF ADRENAL HORMONES

■ The steroid hormones secreted by the adrenal cortex are derived from cholesterol, which is either taken up by the cells from circulating lipoproteins, or synthesized in the cells from acetate.

- Steroid hormones result from a series of biochemical conversions that are performed by enzymes, mainly cytochrome P-450 enzymes in the smooth endoplasmic reticulum and mitochondria.

- The specific steroids produced by each zone of the adrenal cortex depend on the relative activity of the enzymes in that zone (Fig. 21-1).

■ The chromaffin cells of the adrenal medulla synthesize, store, and release catecholamines (i.e., epinephrine, norepinephrine, and dopamine) (Fig. 21-2).

- Most chromaffin cells outside the adrenal medulla lack the enzyme phenylethanolamine-N-methyltransferase, and therefore can make norepinephrine but not epinephrine.

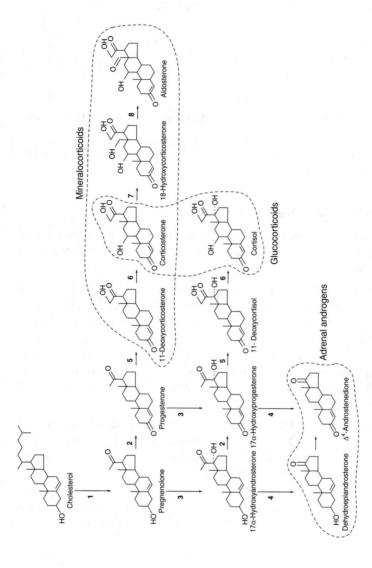

Figure 21-1. Synthesis of steroid hormones in the adrenal cortex. Side-chain cleavage of cholesterol is followed by a series of hydroxylations and other changes to produce the individual steroids. Localization of specific enzymes in areas of the adrenal cortex determines the site of production (e.g., aldosterone synthase in the zona glomerulosa promotes aldosterone production, and 21-hydroxylase in the zona fasciculata promotes cortisol production). The final three steps in the synthesis of aldosterone—11β-hydroxylation, 18-hydroxylation, and 18-methyl oxidation—are catalyzed by a single enzyme, aldosterone synthase. (*1* = cholesterol side-chain cleavage enzyme; *2* = 3β-hydroxysteroid dehydrogenase; *3* = 17α-hydroxylase; *4* = 17,20-lyase; *5* = 21-hydroxylase; *6* = 11β-hydroxylase; *7* = 18-hydroxylase; *8* = 18-methyl oxidase.)

Figure 21-2. Biosynthesis of catecholamines. (*TH* = tyrosine hydroxylase; *AAD* = aromatic-L-amino acid decarboxylase; *DBH* = dopamine-beta-hydroxylase; *PNMT* = phenyleth-anolamine-N-methyltransferase.)

ACTIONS OF ADRENAL HORMONES

🔑 **Cortisol and other glucocorticoids have multiple actions that affect virtually all body tissues. Their main actions are summarized in Table 21-1.**

■ Glucocorticoids, like other steroid hormones, enter cells by passive diffusion and bind to steroid receptors in the cytoplasm or nucleus. The steroid–receptor complex binds to chromosomal DNA and leads to RNA transcription and protein synthesis.

• Some actions of cortisol, such as its effects on growth and on the maintenance of blood pressure, are poorly understood and can only be inferred from the changes observed with cortisol excess or deficiency.

For example, the role of cortisol in resistance to stress is ill defined but crucial: in the absence of enough cortisol, even with adequate mineralocorticoid levels, hypotension, shock, and death may occur.

Possible mechanisms for cortisol's protective effect in stress include its support of cardiovascular function and inhibition of mediators of inflammation and immune response.

Table 21-1. Actions of Glucocorticoids

Intermediary Metabolism

Carbohydrate

  Increased hepatic gluconeogenesis, utilizing amino acids released from muscle and glycerol released from fat

  Inhibition of glucose uptake and metabolism in peripheral tissues

Protein

  Increased protein breakdown, decreased protein synthesis

Fat

  Increased lipolysis

  Redistribution of adipose tissue to head, neck, trunk

Immunologic and Inflammatory Responses

Inhibition of inflammatory agents (e.g., prostaglandins, kinins, histamine)

Redistribution of leukocytes:

  Decrease in circulating lymphocytes, monocytes, and eosinophils

  Increase in circulating polymorphonuclear leukocytes

Suppression of lymphocytes and lymphoid tissue

Cardiovascular System

Support and maintenance of the circulation (hypotension with cortisol deficiency; hypertension with cortisol excess)

Bone, Calcium Metabolism

Negative calcium balance (decreased gastrointestinal absorption, increased renal excretion)

Decreased bone formation, increased resorption

Central Nervous System Effects

Alteration of mood, behavior by either excess or deficiency of cortisol

Growth and Development

Inhibition of growth by cortisol excess

Resistance to Stress

Aldosterone and other mineralocorticoids exert their main effects on the kidneys, in the distal and collecting tubules.

■ Mineralocorticoids increase the reabsorption of filtered sodium by the distal nephron. They increase the permeability of the luminal surface of the tubule cells and stimulate sodium–potassium adenosine triphosphatase (Na,K-ATPase), which pumps sodium from the cell into the interstitial tissues and bloodstream.

• The reabsorption of sodium causes an increase in the electronegativity of the lumen, leading to passive diffusion of potassium into the lumen. The result is sodium retention and potassium excretion.

Catecholamines bind to α-adrenergic and β-adrenergic receptors on the cell surface, and influence many functions in virtually all body tissues.

■ Catecholamines stimulate cardiac rate and force of contraction; increase blood pressure; increase serum glucose levels (due to both increased hepatic glucose production and decreased peripheral glucose utilization); and increase lipolysis and thermogenesis.

CONTROL OF ADRENAL HORMONE PRODUCTION

The synthesis and secretion of cortisol (and the sex steroids of the zona reticularis) are controlled by pituitary ACTH, which in turn depends on hypothalamic corticotropin-releasing hormone (CRH).

■ CRH production depends on three factors: an inborn circadian rhythm (production peaks in early morning, and falls to a nadir at about midnight); the level of stress affecting the individual (communicated by the higher cortical centers); and negative-feedback effects of circulating cortisol (Fig. 21-3).

• Under basal, unstressed conditions, about 10 to 20 mg of cortisol are secreted daily, but the rate rises tenfold with maximal stress.

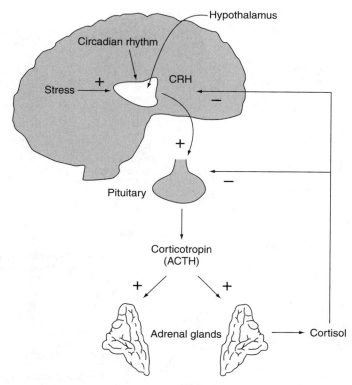

Figure 21-3. The hypothalamic–pituitary–adrenal axis. The negative-feedback effects of cortisol act at both the hypothalamic and pituitary levels.

🔑 **Aldosterone synthesis and secretion are affected by ACTH, but are controlled mainly by the renin–angiotensin system (Fig. 21-4).**

■ A decrease in effective arterial volume triggers renin release. The ensuing increase in angiotensin II-stimulated aldosterone causes sodium and water retention, tending to raise the effective arterial volume toward normal.

   • Also, an increase in serum potassium directly stimulates aldosterone production, increasing renal excretion of potassium.

   • Conditions that may trigger renin and subsequent aldosterone production (secondary hyperaldosteronism) include the following:

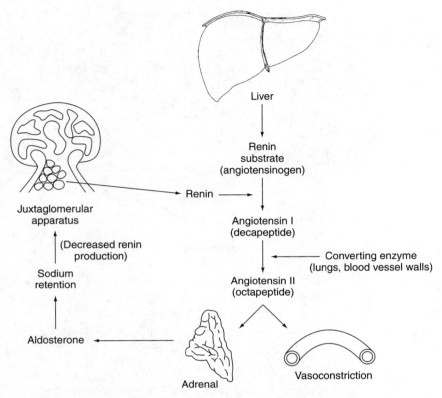

Figure 21-4. The renin–angiotensin system. The juxtaglomerular cells in the afferent arterioles proximal to the renal glomeruli respond to changes in extracellular fluid volume, as indicated by changes in intravascular pressure or stretch of the vessel wall. A decrease in volume triggers renin release, which leads to sodium retention, tending to correct the volume deficit. Conversely, an increase in extracellular volume inhibits renin production, which tends to decrease the volume toward normal.

Decreased vascular volume due to salt restriction, dehydration, or hemorrhage

Movement of fluid from the vascular compartment, as in cirrhosis or nephrotic syndrome

Decreased effective arterial volume due to pump failure, as in congestive heart failure

Decreased pressure or volume sensing by the renal juxtaglomerular cells, as in renovascular or malignant hypertension

The production and release of catecholamines by the adrenal medulla is controlled by neural impulses from the central nervous system.

■ Tracts descend from the medulla, pons, and hypothalamus, and synapse in the intermediolateral cell column of the spinal cord with preganglionic fibers that make up the splanchnic nerves to the adrenal medulla.

• The sympathetic impulses that trigger catecholamine release may be initiated by many factors, including baroreceptor reflexes, metabolic changes such as hypoglycemia or anoxia, or stress ("fight or flight" response).

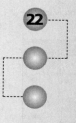

Adrenal Insufficiency

Inadequate adrenal production of cortisol and aldosterone produces important physiologic derangements, which, when severe, are incompatible with life. Replacement of cortisol and treatment with an aldosterone-like steroid can reverse the abnormalities of adrenal insufficiency, but the dosage of cortisol must be adjusted carefully at times of stress.

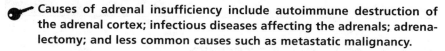

CAUSES AND MANIFESTATIONS OF ADRENAL INSUFFICIENCY

🔑 **Causes of adrenal insufficiency include autoimmune destruction of the adrenal cortex; infectious diseases affecting the adrenals; adrenalectomy; and less common causes such as metastatic malignancy.**

■ Autoimmune destruction of the adrenal cortex is the most common cause of primary adrenal insufficiency (Addison's disease).

- Infectious diseases, including tuberculosis, fungal diseases, and syphilis, may involve and destroy the adrenals.

- Acquired immunodeficiency syndrome (AIDS) and its infectious complications, especially cytomegalovirus, are also important causes of Addison's disease.

- Iatrogenic adrenal insufficiency results from bilateral adrenalectomy.

- Long-term suppression of adrenal function may follow prolonged glucocorticoid therapy.

- Less common causes of adrenal insufficiency include bilateral adrenal hemorrhage, amyloidosis, metastatic malignancy or lymphoma, and adrenoleukodystrophy.

■ Secondary adrenal insufficiency results from deficient adrenocorticotropic hormone (ACTH) production by the pituitary gland (see Chapter 2).

■ Manifestations of adrenal insufficiency are shown in Table 22-1.

- Hyperpigmentation of the skin is caused by melanocyte-stimulating hormone (MSH), which is part of the ACTH-precursor molecule proopiomelanocortin (POMC).

    POMC is produced in response to negative feedback from the low circulating cortisol levels.

Table 22-1. Manifestations of Adrenal Insufficiency

Cortisol Deficiency	Aldosterone Deficiency

Hyperpigmentation of skin and mucous membranes	Sodium loss:
	  Hyponatremia
	  Hypovolemia, weight loss
	  Decreased cardiac output, hypotension
	  Decreased renal blood flow, azotemia

Hypotension, postural or sustained	
Hypoglycemia	

GI: anorexia, nausea, vomiting	Potassium retention:
	  Hyperkalemia
	  Cardiac arrhythmias

CNS: lethargy, confusion, psychiatric symptoms	
Arthralgias, myalgias	
Inability to tolerate stress	

DIAGNOSIS OF ADRENAL INSUFFICIENCY

The diagnosis of adrenal insufficiency may be suggested by the findings in Table 22-1, especially darkening of the skin or the combination of hyponatremia and hyperkalemia. Definitive diagnosis is made by showing that adrenal production of cortisol does not respond to the injection of ACTH, as it does in normal persons.

- In the standard ACTH test, 25 to 40 units of ACTH are infused intravenously (IV) for 8 hours.

  - A normal response to the standard test is a threefold to fivefold increase in the 24-hour urinary excretion of corticoids (metabolites of cortisol) or an increase in serum cortisol of 15 to 40 µg/dL.

- A short version of the ACTH test is commonly performed. A single intramuscular or intravenous injection of 25 units of ACTH is given, and plasma cortisol is measured 30 or 60 minutes later.

  - Cortisol normally reaches a level of 20 µg/dL or higher in response to ACTH.

- Inadequate cortisol response to ACTH does not differentiate between primary (Addison's disease) or secondary (pituitary) adrenal insufficiency, because prolonged lack of ACTH stimulation may cause the adrenals to be suppressed and unable to respond rapidly to ACTH.

  - Inadequate ACTH production, rather than primary adrenal disease, is indicated to be the primary cause by the following findings.

Baseline serum ACTH levels are low rather than high.

Continued ACTH administration for several days is followed by eventual, although not initial, adrenal response (a "priming" effect).

TREATMENT OF ADRENAL INSUFFICIENCY

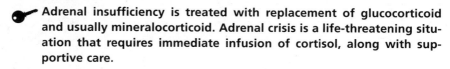 **Adrenal insufficiency is treated with replacement of glucocorticoid and usually mineralocorticoid. Adrenal crisis is a life-threatening situation that requires immediate infusion of cortisol, along with supportive care.**

■ Glucocorticoid replacement is achieved with oral cortisol (hydrocortisone), typically 20 mg each morning with or without an additional 10 mg in the evening.

  • The usual dose must be doubled or tripled with minor stress (e.g., an upper respiratory infection), and increased up to tenfold with severe stress (e.g., major illness, surgery, or trauma).

■ Mineralocorticoid replacement is needed in most patients with primary adrenal insufficiency, but not in those with secondary adrenal insufficiency because the renin–angiotensin–aldosterone axis is not affected.

  • Fludrocortisone (Florinef) is a synthetic steroid with almost pure mineralocorticoid activity; it is used in doses of 50 to 200 µg daily (aldosterone is not available as a pharmacologic agent).

  • Hypotension (despite adequate cortisol replacement) or persistent hyponatremia, hyperkalemia, or weakness may indicate the need for more mineralocorticoid.

  • Hypertension, edema, hypernatremia, or hypokalemia may indicate a need for less mineralocorticoid replacement.

■ Adrenal crisis is an acute life-threatening exacerbation of adrenal insufficiency that is marked by fever, abdominal pain, vomiting, altered mental status, and vascular collapse.

  • Adrenal crisis is treated with immediate intravenous infusion of 100 mg of cortisol, followed by stress doses of cortisol (300 mg daily).

    Supportive measures include IV administration of saline and mineralocorticoid, if necessary.

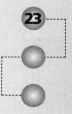

Cushing's Syndrome

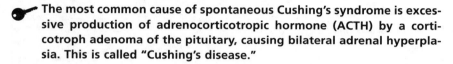

Cushing's syndrome is a condition caused by excessive circulating levels of cortisol or other glucocorticoid hormone. The hypercortisolism may be caused by disorders of the pituitary or adrenal glands, by tumors that make ACTH, or by prolonged use of glucocorticoids as anti-inflammatory or immunosuppressive agents in the treatment of certain diseases.

CAUSES AND MANIFESTATIONS OF CUSHING'S SYNDROME

The most common cause of spontaneous Cushing's syndrome is excessive production of adrenocorticotropic hormone (ACTH) by a corticotroph adenoma of the pituitary, causing bilateral adrenal hyperplasia. This is called "Cushing's disease."

- Tumors that secrete excess cortisol or produce ACTH abnormally are other causes of Cushing's syndrome.

  - Cushing's syndrome is caused by adrenal tumors, either adenomas or carcinomas, that secrete excess cortisol.

  - Ectopic ACTH production by malignant tumors such as oat cell lung cancer, carcinoma of the pancreas, or bronchial carcinoid tumors also causes Cushing's syndrome.

    "Ectopic" refers to production of a hormone by a tissue that does not normally produce that hormone.

- Manifestations of Cushing's syndrome are shown in Table 23-1 and Figure 23-1.

  - The hypertension probably is caused by both the direct vascular effects and the weak mineralocorticoid effects of cortisol.

  - Adrenal androgens may be overproduced in addition to cortisol, explaining the androgenic manifestations.

  - Other manifestations may be related to the catabolic effects of cortisol on bone, muscle, and skin, and direct effects on the central nervous system.

Table 23-1. Manifestations of Cushing's Syndrome

"Cushingoid" changes in appearance:

    Central obesity (fat accumulation in face, neck, trunk; "moon face"; "buffalo hump"; supraclavicular fat pads; extremities remain thin)

    Purple striae

    Facial plethora

    Easy bruising

Hypertension

Decreased glucose tolerance

    Overt diabetes in 20%

Androgen excess in women

    Menstrual abnormalities

    Hirsutism

    Acne

Muscle wasting, weakness

Osteoporosis

Depression; other psychiatric disturbances

Growth retardation in children

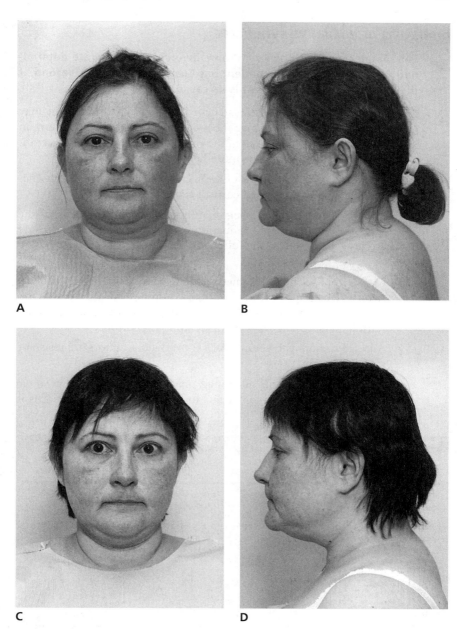

A

B

C

D

Figure 23-1. A 47-year-old woman with Cushing's syndrome caused by an adrenal adenoma. (*A, B*) Central obesity ("moon face"), facial plethora, and a dorsal fat pad ("buffalo hump") are evident in photographs taken before surgery. (*C,D*) Nine months after removal of the adrenal tumor, the patient has lost 20 pounds, the plethora is no longer present, and the dorsal fat pad has decreased in size.

DIAGNOSIS OF CUSHING'S SYNDROME

 The diagnosis of Cushing's syndrome involves two separate determinations: first, whether the patient has Cushing's syndrome; second, if the syndrome is present, what is its cause.

- Serum cortisol levels are elevated in Cushing's syndrome, but may overlap with the normal range. Loss of the normal diurnal pattern, in which cortisol reaches a peak in the early morning and then falls gradually until midnight, may be more helpful in diagnosis.
  - The most useful indicator of daily cortisol secretion is determination of 24-hour urine free cortisol excretion.
- Because baseline cortisol levels may not be diagnostic, tests of the suppressibility of cortisol production often are needed (Table 23-2.) These tests are based on the following observations.
  - Production of ACTH by the normal hypothalamic–pituitary axis is easily suppressed by dexamethasone (a potent synthetic glucocorticoid). This is not true in Cushing's syndrome. For this reason, the response to a low dose of dexamethasone may distinguish between normal persons and those with Cushing's syndrome.
  - Adrenal tumors and ectopic ACTH-producing tumors are resistant to suppression.
  - Pituitary corticotroph adenomas may be suppressed, but their threshold for suppression seems to be raised: ACTH and cortisol

Table 23-2. Dexamethasone Suppression Tests for Cushing's Syndrome			
	Dose of Dexamethasone	Serum Cortisol Measurement	Normal Response
Short (overnight) low-dose test	1.0 mg at 11 P.M.	8 A.M. the following day	Serum cortisol <3.0 µg/dL
Standard low-dose test	0.5 mg every 6 hours for 8 doses, starting 8 A.M.	8 A.M. after last dose	Serum cortisol <2.0 µg/dL
Overnight high-dose test	8 mg at 11 P.M. on day 1	8 A.M. on days 1 and 2	>50% fall in serum cortisol on day 2
Standard high-dose test	2.0 mg every 6 hours for 8 doses, starting 8 A.M.	Baseline, and 8 A.M. after last dose	>50% fall in serum cortisol

production are lowered by high doses of dexamethasone, but not by the low doses that suppress the normal hypothalamic–pituitary–adrenal axis.

For this reason, the response to a high dose of dexamethasone may distinguish between patients with a corticotroph adenoma, who respond, and those with an adrenal tumor or ectopic ACTH production, who do not respond.

• The overnight low-dose dexamethasone suppression test is an efficient screening test for Cushing's syndrome, followed by urine free cortisol measurements, if indicated (Fig. 23-2A).

In equivocal cases, the standard low-dose suppression test may be combined with an injection of corticotropin-releasing

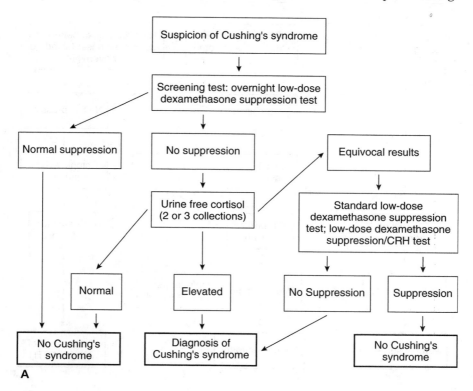

Figure 23-2. Algorithms for diagnosis of Cushing's syndrome. (*A*) Making the diagnosis of Cushing's syndrome. (Adapted from MYERS AR: *Medicine, 4th ed.* Philadelphia, J. B. Lippincott Company, 2001, p. 535.)

hormone (CRH), which has an overly stimulatory effect on corticotroph adenomas and therefore may exaggerate their failure to be suppressed normally.

■ If Cushing's syndrome is diagnosed, additional studies may help to pinpoint the cause (Fig. 23-2B).

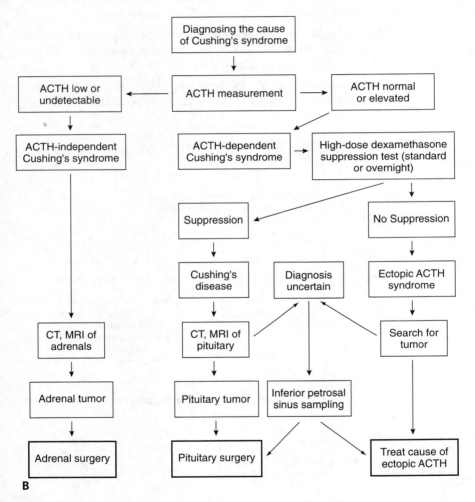

Figure 23-2. Continued (B) Ascertaining the specific cause of Cushing's syndrome. (Adapted from MYERS AR: *Medicine, 4th ed.* Philadelphia, J. B. Lippincott Company, 2001, p. 535.)

- Serum ACTH levels will be suppressed by the autonomous cortisol production of an adrenal tumor (ACTH-independent Cushing's syndrome), but will be high-normal or elevated in patients with corticotroph adenomas or ectopic ACTH production (ACTH-dependent Cushing's syndrome).

- Bilateral sampling of blood from the inferior petrosal sinuses, which drain the pituitary area, will reveal increased ACTH concentrations relative to peripheral blood in patients with corticotroph adenomas, but not in those with ectopic ACTH production. Injection of CRH may magnify these differences.

- Computed tomographic (CT) scan and magnetic resonance imaging (MRI) of the adrenals and pituitary may reveal tumors of those glands.

TREATMENT OF CUSHING'S SYNDROME

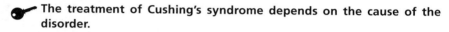 **The treatment of Cushing's syndrome depends on the cause of the disorder.**

- Surgical removal of adrenal adenomas that produce excess cortisol will cure the Cushing's syndrome. Replacement therapy with cortisol is needed until the remaining adrenal gland, which has been suppressed by prolonged cortisol excess, regains normal function.

- Adrenal carcinoma often has metastasized by the time the diagnosis is made, and the tumors that cause ectopic ACTH production may not be curable.

  - In these patients, drugs that directly inhibit adrenal production of cortisol may be used to relieve the manifestations of hypercortisolism even though the cortisol-producing tissue cannot be removed.

    These drugs include mitotane, metyrapone, aminoglutethimide, and ketoconazole.

- Cushing's disease is usually treated with transsphenoidal pituitary surgery: the corticotroph adenoma is removed successfully in 50% to 95% of cases.

  - Pituitary irradiation alone is often effective in curing Cushing's disease in children, but is less successful in adults.

  - Bilateral adrenalectomy will cure the Cushing's disease, but the patient is left with Addison's disease that requires lifelong treatment.

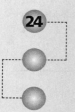

Primary Aldosteronism

Increased aldosterone production commonly occurs when extracellular fluid volume is depleted; it is considered a *secondary* phenomenon because it occurs in response to physiologic changes and tends to restore homeostasis. *Primary* hyperaldosteronism, in contrast, is caused by disease of the adrenal cortex; the inappropriate excess of mineralocorticoid activity causes hypertension and other manifestations.

CAUSES AND MANIFESTATIONS OF PRIMARY ALDOSTERONISM

Primary oversecretion of aldosterone commonly is caused by a small (0.5 to 3.0 cm) adrenal adenoma, but in 20% to 40% of cases there is bilateral hyperplasia of the adrenal cortex.

■ The reabsorption of sodium and water that occurs in response to hyperaldosteronism leads to expansion of extracellular fluid volume. Compensatory changes in renal hemodynamics and natriuretic hormones limit the retention of salt and water to 1 to 2 kg before a new equilibrium is reached.

• This amount of volume expansion usually does not cause edema, but the increase in cardiac output, and perhaps other factors, causes hypertension.

• Hyperaldosteronism also causes urinary loss of potassium, which may result in hypokalemia.

Severe hypokalemia may be manifested by muscle weakness and by vacuolar nephropathy of the distal tubules; the latter may cause polyuria due to nephrogenic diabetes insipidus.

DIAGNOSIS OF PRIMARY ALDOSTERONISM

The key to the diagnosis of primary aldosteronism is the finding of increased aldosterone production in the presence of *low*, rather than *high*, plasma renin activity (Fig. 24-1).

■ This occurs because the various causes of secondary aldosteronism, which is far more common than primary aldosteronism, stimulate renin, which in turn stimulates angiotensin II and aldosterone; in primary aldosteronism, the hyperaldosteronism causes suppression of renin production.

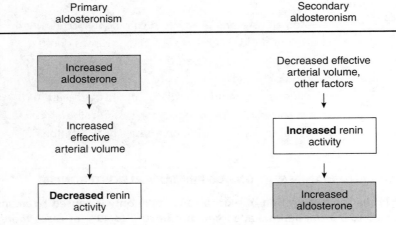

Figure 24-1. The sequence of events causing primary aldosteronism, contrasted with the sequence of events in secondary aldosteronism. This explains why the combination of increased aldosterone and decreased renin activity is pathognomonic for primary aldosteronism.

- If hypertension and hypokalemia raise the suspicion of primary aldosteronism, the best initial test is the simultaneous measurement, with the patient in the upright position, of serum aldosterone and plasma renin activity.
  - If the aldosterone:renin ratio (ng/dL:ng AII/mL/h) is greater than 25, further study is indicated (Fig. 24-2).
- Aldosterone excess is demonstrated most convincingly by failure to suppress aldosterone by volume expansion.
  - A serum aldosterone level that is greater than 10 ng/dL after a 4-hour infusion of 2000 mL of normal saline indicates hyperaldosteronism.
- Alternatively, a 24-hour urine may be collected after oral salt loading for 3 days (10 to 12 g of added salt per day).
  - Urinary aldosterone greater than 10 to 14 μg/24 hours indicates failure of suppression, provided adequate salt loading is confirmed by a urine sodium level greater than 250 mmol/24 hours.

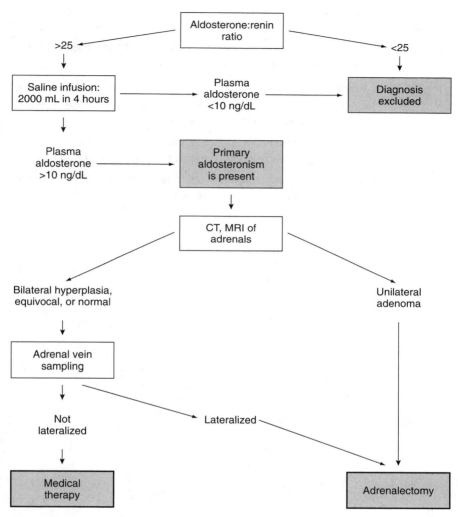

Figure 24-2. Algorithm for the diagnosis of primary aldosteronism.

TREATMENT OF PRIMARY ALDOSTERONISM

 Primary aldosteronism may be treated surgically or with medical therapy, with improvement or relief of symptoms.

- An aldosterone-producing adenoma is treated by surgical removal.
  - The hypertension is cured or improved in most cases, but persists in some. The hypokalemia is almost always relieved.
- Primary hyperaldosteronism caused by bilateral adrenal hyperplasia is usually not cured by surgery, and medical therapy is preferable.
  - Spironolactone, which inhibits the actions of aldosterone on the renal tubules, is the medical treatment of choice.

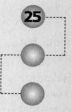

Pheochromocytoma

Pheochromocytoma is a rare tumor that arises from chromaffin cells, which are located mainly in the adrenal medulla but are also in sympathetic ganglia and elsewhere. The tumor causes hypertension and other manifestations of catecholamine hormone excess.

ETIOLOGY AND MANIFESTATIONS OF PHEOCHROMOCYTOMA

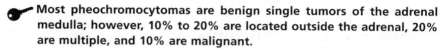 **Most pheochromocytomas are benign single tumors of the adrenal medulla; however, 10% to 20% are located outside the adrenal, 20% are multiple, and 10% are malignant.**

■ The manifestations of pheochromocytoma are listed in Table 25-1.

• The finding that is most suggestive of a pheochromocytoma is the occurrence of paroxysmal episodes, lasting less than an hour, of increased blood pressure and hyperadrenergic symptoms.

Table 25-1. Manifestations of Pheochromocytoma
Hypertension
Paroxysmal in 50%
Sustained in 50%
Headache
Sweating
Palpitations
Nervousness, tremor
Hypermetabolism and weight loss
Hyperglycemia
Postural hypotension (despite supine hypertension)

DIAGNOSIS OF PHEOCHROMOCYTOMA

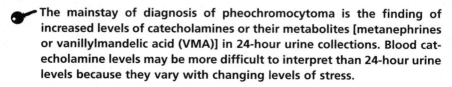 **The mainstay of diagnosis of pheochromocytoma is the finding of increased levels of catecholamines or their metabolites [metanephrines or vanillylmandelic acid (VMA)] in 24-hour urine collections. Blood catecholamine levels may be more difficult to interpret than 24-hour urine levels because they vary with changing levels of stress.**

■ If increased catecholamine levels suggest a pheochromocytoma but are not diagnostic, a clonidine-suppression test may be useful.

• An oral dose of 0.3 mg clonidine causes elevated catecholamine levels to fall to normal within 3 hours if they are elevated because of stress, but does not significantly affect catecholamine levels that are elevated because of a pheochromocytoma.

■ Pheochromocytomas are usually large enough to be visualized by computed tomographic (CT) scans or magnetic resonance imaging (MRI). Isotope scanning with ^{131}I-iodobenzylguanidine (MIBG) may reveal extra-adrenal as well as adrenal tumors.

TREATMENT OF PHEOCHROMOCYTOMA

🔑 **Surgical removal of the pheochromocytoma is the treatment of choice.**

■ Vascular instability and shock may occur when the source of excessive catecholamines is suddenly removed.

• These patients may have accommodated to long-term adrenergic stimulation with down-regulation of adrenergic receptors, leaving them less responsive to the lower concentrations of circulating catecholamines. Also, they may have decreased blood volume since the vascular compartment is contracted because of vasoconstriction of capacitance vessels.

• Pretreatment with α-adrenergic receptor blockers lessens the risk of vascular instability and shock.

• If tachycardia or another arrhythmia is present, β-blockers also may be used.

α-Adrenergic receptor blockers include phenoxybenzamine, phentolamine, and the newer drugs prazosin, terazosin, and doxazosin.

β-Adrenergic receptor blockers should not be used alone, because unopposed α-adrenergic stimulation may worsen the hypertension, but they may be used with α-adrenergic blockers.

Female Reproduction

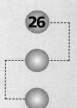

26   The Ovaries

The ovaries provide a mature ovum, capable of being fertilized, at regular intervals during the reproductive years between puberty and menopause. The ovaries also produce the hormones estrogen and progesterone, which affect the monthly cycle, secondary sexual characteristics, and other functions. Disorders that affect the ovaries may interfere with ovulation and menstruation, causing infertility, and may affect many functions through alterations in the circulating levels of estrogen, androgens, and progesterone.

OVARIAN MORPHOLOGY

 The ovary consists of an outer area or cortex that contains the ovarian follicles, and an inner area or medulla that contains connective tissue cells and interstitial secretory cells (i.e., the stroma). The hilus of the ovary is its point of attachment to the mesentery and the entrance of blood vessels and nerves.

■ Most ovarian follicles are small, nongrowing *primordial* follicles that consist of a small oocyte arrested in early meiosis and a single layer of future granulosa cells.

   • When a primordial follicle starts to grow, it progresses through stages in which it is called a *primary follicle,* then a *secondary follicle,* and ultimately a *preovulatory* or *Graafian follicle.*

      In this process the oocyte enlarges, the granulosa cell layer expands, and stromal cells differentiate to form layers of cells called the *theca interna* and *theca externa.*

      An internal cavity, the antrum, forms in the granulosa cell layer. The antrum is filled with follicular fluid and causes the oocyte to occupy an eccentric position in the follicle (Fig. 26-1).

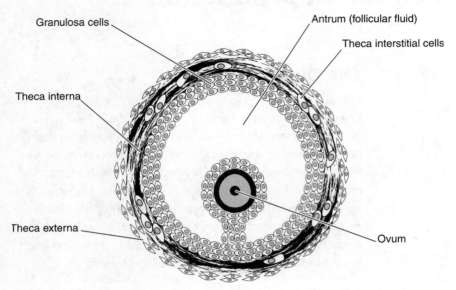

Granulosa cells

Antrum (follicular fluid)

Theca interstitial cells

Theca interna

Theca externa

Ovum

Figure 26-1. Drawing of a Graafian follicle, showing the location of the ovum, the granulosa cell layer, and the theca interna and externa.

OVARIAN HORMONES

 The steroid hormones produced by the ovary are estrogens (estradiol and estrone), progesterone, and androgens (androstenedione and testosterone).

■ The main function of ovarian androgens is to act as substrate for estrogen production: estradiol is formed by the aromatization of testosterone, and estrone is formed by the aromatization of androstenedione (Fig. 26-2).

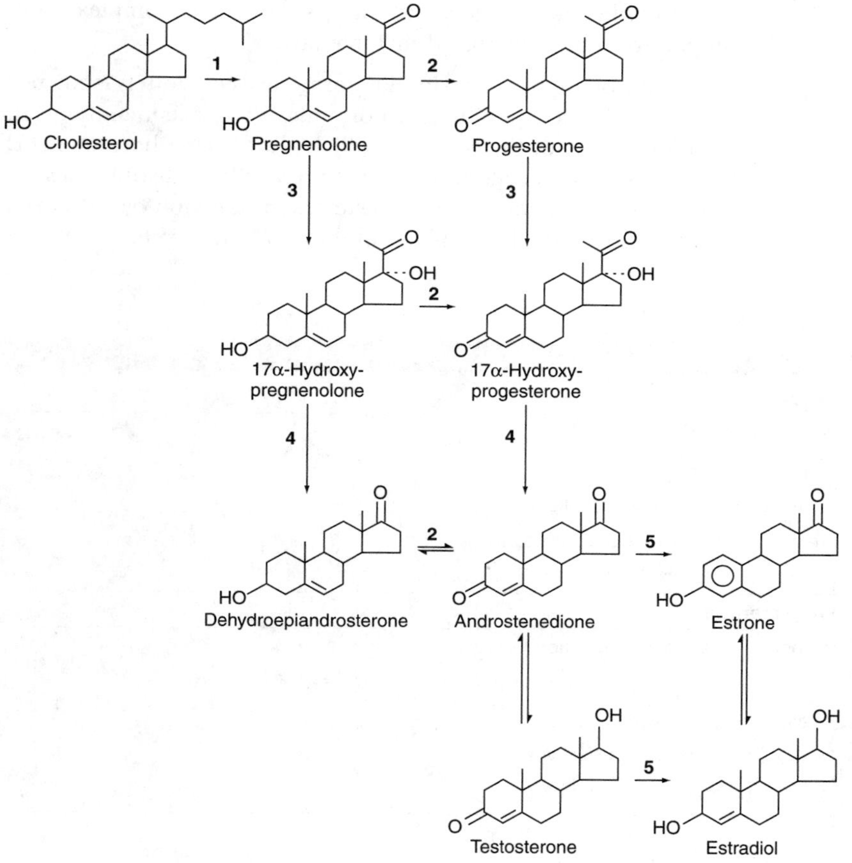

Figure 26-2. Biosynthesis of steroids in the ovary. (*1* = cholesterol side-chain cleavage enzyme; *2* = 3β-hydroxysteroid dehydrogenase; *3* = 17α-hydroxylase; *4* = 17, 20-lyase; *5* = aromatase; *6* = 17α-hydroxysteroid dehydrogenase.)

- The actions of estrogen and progesterone are complex; some important actions are listed in Table 26-1.

- The control of ovarian steroid hormone secretion is shown in Fig. 26-3. Follicle-stimulating hormone (FSH) acts mainly on the granulosa cells of the Graafian follicle; luteinizing hormone (LH) acts on the thecal cells and the granulosa cells, and stimulates corpus luteum formation and progesterone production by the corpus luteum during the luteal phase of the menstrual cycle.

Table 26-1. Actions of Ovarian Steroid Hormones

Estrogen

Proliferation of granulosa cells in ovary

Proliferation of endometrial cells

Proliferation of vaginal epithelium

Breast development: ducts, adipose tissue

Metabolic effects on liver, plasma lipids, bone, kidney

Progesterone

Inhibition of estrogen production in ovary

Decrease in proliferation of endometrium, induction of secretory phase

Breast: formation of secretory alveoli

Metabolic effects on plasma lipids

Increase in basal body temperature

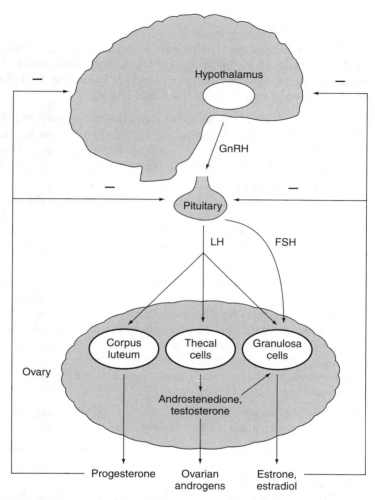

Figure 26-3. The control of ovarian steroid hormone production. Although ovarian steroid hormones generally have negative feedback effects on the hypothalamus and pituitary, in certain circumstances increased estrogen levels are thought to stimulate pituitary secretion of LH (as in the latter part of the follicular phase of the menstrual cycle, and in the polycystic ovary syndrome).

THE MENSTRUAL CYCLE

 The typical menstrual cycle of 28 days is depicted in Figure 26-4. The onset of menstrual bleeding marks day 1, and ovulation typically occurs on day 14. The first half of the cycle is known as the follicular phase; the second half is called the luteal phase.

- Each month, 5 to 15 follicles in the primordial or primary stage begin to mature rapidly. During the second half of the follicular phase, one follicle becomes dominant and continues to mature into a Graafian follicle, while the other follicles stop growing and undergo atresia.

- Estrogen, produced by the follicular cells of the rapidly growing dominant follicle, increases in serum concentration through the follicular phase of the cycle. The rising estrogen level exerts a positive feedback effect on pituitary production of LH; this, along with increased secretion of gonadotropin-releasing hormone (GnRH) by the hypothalamus, produces a midcycle surge of LH.

- The LH surge causes ovulation, which is the rupture of the Graafian follicle with extrusion of the ovum. LH then causes the ruptured follicle to form a corpus luteum; "luteinization" of the follicular and thecal cells occurs, with lipid droplet formation and changes in the mitochondria and endoplasmic reticulum. The corpus luteum, stimulated by LH, produces progesterone during the luteal phase of the cycle, and then undergoes lysis and transformation into the scar-like corpus albicans.

  - Basal body temperature rises 0.5° F to 1.0° F during the luteal phase through a direct effect of progesterone on thermoregulation.

- The endometrium proliferates under the influence of estrogen during the follicular phase of the cycle, and becomes more vascular, with coiled, secretory glands, under the influence of progesterone in the luteal phase. When the corpus luteum undergoes lysis at the end of the cycle, with a fall in estrogen and progesterone levels, endometrial blood vessels undergo necrosis and the uterine lining is shed during menstruation.

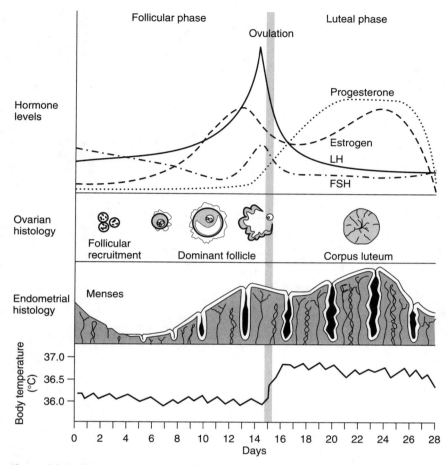

Figure 26-4. Diagrammatic representation of the menstrual cycle, showing the changes in hormone levels, ovarian follicle development, endometrial histology, and basal body temperature during the cycle.

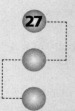

Amenorrhea

Endocrine disorders that affect the female reproductive system frequently cause amenorrhea or other changes in the menstrual cycle.

CAUSES OF AMENORRHEA

🔑 **Amenorrhea refers to the failure to undergo menarche by age 16 (primary amenorrhea), or cessation of menstrual periods for more than 3 months in a previously menstruating woman (secondary amenorrhea).**

- Primary amenorrhea may be caused by abnormalities of the ovaries, pituitary, or adrenals, or by structural abnormalities of the genital tract (Table 27-1).

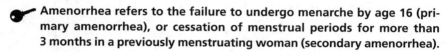

Table 27-1. Causes of Primary Amenorrhea
Gonadal causes
Gonadal dysgenesis (Turner's syndrome)
Testicular feminization syndrome
Resistant ovary syndrome
Extragonadal causes
Panhypopituitarism
Hypogonadotropic hypogonadism
Delayed menarche
Congenital adrenal hyperplasia
Abnormalities of uterus or vagina

- Secondary amenorrhea may be physiologic (e.g., pregnancy, menopause) or may reflect endocrine or structural disorders (Table 27-2).

Table 27-2. Causes of Secondary Amenorrhea

Pregnancy

Menopause

Uterine causes (e.g., hysterectomy, inflammatory disorders)

Hypothalamic–pituitary causes

  Hypopituitarism

  Hypothalamic ("psychogenic") amenorrhea

  Malnutrition, chronic illness

  Physical training

  Discontinuation of oral contraceptives

Ovarian causes

  Primary ovarian failure ("premature menopause")

  Oophorectomy, radiotherapy, chemotherapy

Estrogen excess: ovarian tumors

Prolactin excess: pituitary tumors, medications

Androgen excess

  Polycystic ovary syndrome

  Overproduction of adrenal androgen

  Ovarian tumors

GONADAL DYSGENESIS (TURNER'S SYNDROME)

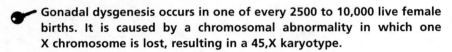

Gonadal dysgenesis occurs in one of every 2500 to 10,000 live female births. It is caused by a chromosomal abnormality in which one X chromosome is lost, resulting in a 45,X karyotype.

- The ovaries fail to develop; in their place are streaks of connective tissue, without ova. Without the major source of estrogen production, the breasts do not develop and other secondary sexual characteristics do not appear.

- Associated somatic abnormalities may include short stature, webbed neck, epicanthal folds, shield-like chest, and abnormalities of the heart and kidneys.

- Estrogen therapy produces secondary sexual characteristics, but not fertility. Growth hormone may be used to increase adult height.

HYPOTHALAMIC AMENORRHEA

Hypothalamic amenorrhea (also called "psychogenic" or "functional" amenorrhea) is the most common cause of secondary amenorrhea. Psychological stress, poor nutrition, or other factors may interfere with the normal pulsatile secretion of gonadotropin-releasing hormone (GnRH) by the hypothalamus.

- Serum levels of luteinizing hormone (LH) and follicle-stimulating hormone (FSH) are normal or low in hypothalamic amenorrhea, and estrogen and progesterone levels may be low because of the absence of follicle development, ovulation, and corpus luteum formation.

- The primary role of hypothalamic dysfunction in most cases of functional or idiopathic amenorrhea is supported by the clinical response to treatment with the hypothalamic hormone GnRH.

  - If GnRH is administered (via infusion pump) in the physiologic pattern of pulse doses every 90 to 120 minutes, normal function may be restored, including ovulation, corpus luteum formation, and subsequent pregnancy.

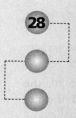

Polycystic Ovary Syndrome

Polycystic ovary syndrome (PCOS) is the most common endocrine disorder in reproductive-age women, with a prevalence of 3% to 7%. The main feature of the syndrome is chronic lack of ovulation, associated with infertility and often with androgen excess, obesity, and insulin resistance.

PATHOPHYSIOLOGY OF POLYCYSTIC OVARY SYNDROME

The ovaries in women with PCOS produce increased amounts of androgens, especially androstenedione (Fig. 28-1.) Conversion of these androgens to estrogens, especially estrone, occurs in fat and other peripheral tissues, so that blood levels of both androstenedione and estrone may be elevated.

■ Positive feedback effects of the increased estrogen levels stimulate luteinizing hormone (LH) production, which in turn may stimulate androgen production by the ovarian thecal cells and stroma. Negative feedback effects of estrogen may inhibit follicle-stimulating hormone

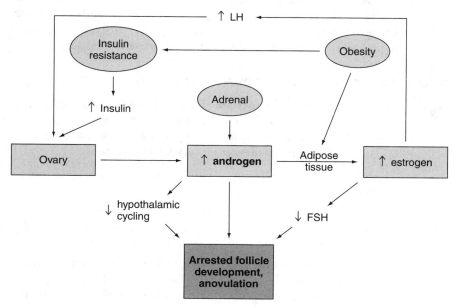

Figure 28-1. Pathogenesis of polycystic ovary syndrome. (Adapted from MYERS AR: *Medicine, 4th ed.* Philadelphia, J. B. Lippincott Company, 2001, p. 536.)

(FSH) production; an elevated LH-to-FSH ratio (>2) is characteristic of PCOS.

- The arrested follicle development and anovulation that are the prime features of PCOS are caused by the decrease in FSH, the elevation in circulating androgens, and the absence of normal cyclic hypothalamic–pituitary control of LH and FSH secretion. The arrested follicle development leads to enlargement of the ovaries, which have thickened capsules, many small follicular cysts on the surface, and stromal and thecal hyperplasia.

■ Insulin resistance, with consequent elevation of serum insulin levels, is common in PCOS.

- The increased insulin levels may contribute to the increased ovarian production of androgens. Drugs that decrease insulin resistance (e.g., metformin, troglitazone) have lowered androgen levels and produced ovulation in some women with PCOS.

- Obesity may contribute to the insulin resistance and to the peripheral conversion of androgen to estrogen. Adrenal overproduction of androgens may contribute to the syndrome in some cases.

■ The primary abnormality responsible for PCOS is not known, and probably differs from patient to patient. Proposed initiating events include insulin resistance, primary ovarian disease, abnormal hypothalamic–pituitary function, and primary adrenal disease.

MANAGEMENT OF POLYCYSTIC OVARY SYNDROME

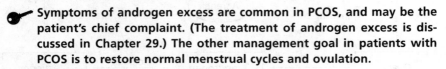 **Symptoms of androgen excess are common in PCOS, and may be the patient's chief complaint. (The treatment of androgen excess is discussed in Chapter 29.) The other management goal in patients with PCOS is to restore normal menstrual cycles and ovulation.**

■ The infertility that results from chronic anovulation may be treated in several ways.

- Clomiphene citrate stimulates LH and FSH production by blocking the binding of estrogen to its receptors and thus inhibiting the negative-feedback effects of estrogen on the pituitary.

- If clomiphene citrate does not restore ovulation, human menopausal gonadotropin (which has FSH and LH activity) and human chorionic gonadotrophin (which has mainly LH activity) may be used in a way that mimics the secretion of gonadotropins during the normal menstrual cycle.

■ Even if pregnancy is not desired, the chronic anovulation and amenorrhea or oligomenorrhea require attention, because constant stimulation of the endometrium by unopposed estrogen may cause functional bleeding and may increase the risk of endometrial cancer.

• A progesterone preparation such as medroxyprogesterone acetate, taken for 10 days every month (or every few months) will interrupt the persistent endometrial proliferation by causing sloughing of the endometrium and bleeding within a few days of completing the course of treatment.

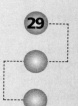

Other Androgen Excess Syndromes

29

Mild elevation of serum androgen levels in women may cause oiliness of the skin, acne, irregular menses, and male-pattern growth of hair on the face and body (i.e., hirsutism). More severe androgen excess can cause true virilization, with deepening of the voice, enlargement of the clitoris, and more masculine body shape and muscle development. Either the ovaries or the adrenal glands may be the source of excess testosterone or androstenedione.

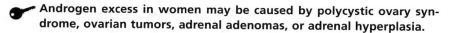

CAUSES OF ANDROGEN EXCESS IN WOMEN

Androgen excess in women may be caused by polycystic ovary syndrome, ovarian tumors, adrenal adenomas, or adrenal hyperplasia.

- Polycystic ovary syndrome (described in Chapter 28) is an important cause of androgen excess.

- Androgen-producing ovarian tumors include arrhenoblastomas, hilar cell tumors, adrenal rest tumors, and granulosa cell tumors.
  - Very high serum testosterone levels and physical findings of virilization suggest an ovarian tumor, which should be sought using pelvic examination and imaging techniques.

- Adrenal adenomas or carcinomas may produce excess androgens. High levels of adrenal androgens, dehydroepiandrosterone (DHEA) and DHEA-sulfate (DHEA-S), which cannot be suppressed by dexamethasone, suggest this diagnosis. (DHEA and DHEA-S are not themselves androgenic, but may be converted to testosterone and androstenedione).

- Congenital adrenal hyperplasia is a genetic defect in one of the enzymes involved in the synthesis of cortisol, most commonly 21β-hydroxylase (see Fig. 21-1).
  - Decreased cortisol synthesis stimulates pituitary adrenocorticotropic hormone (ACTH) production, which causes adrenal growth and increased activity of the cortisol synthetic pathway so that adequate cortisol is made despite the enzyme defect. But this adrenal stimulation also leads to increased production of adrenal androgens by the zona reticularis, and the result is androgen excess.

- If manifested during fetal development or childhood, this defect can cause pseudohermaphroditism or virilization in girls and premature pubertal changes in boys. However, the first manifestations are often androgen excess symptoms in young adult women; the diagnosis may be suggested by an elevated level of 17-OH-progesterone, the precursor of the defective 21-hydroxylation step in cortisol synthesis (see Fig. 21-1).

- Specific treatment of congenital adrenal hyperplasia is administration of a glucocorticoid, which will suppress ACTH and reverse the process that led to androgen excess.

■ "Idiopathic hirsutism" is a poorly defined but common disorder in which hirsutism may exist without other manifestations of androgen excess, with or without elevated androgen levels, and without evident cause.

- In patients with normal androgen levels, an increase in the sensitivity of hair follicles to androgen stimulation is postulated.

MANAGEMENT OF ANDROGEN-EXCESS DISORDERS

🔑 **Specific measures have been discussed for the management of the polycystic ovary syndrome and congenital adrenal hyperplasia. Ovarian and adrenal tumors may be surgically removed.**

■ Idiopathic hirsutism, or hirsutism associated with other androgenic disorders, may be treated in several ways.

- Mechanical methods of hair control include shaving, electrolysis, laser therapy, bleaching, chemical depilatories, and wax treatments.

- Spironolactone, an aldosterone antagonist used mainly in hypertension and disorders causing fluid retention, also decreases androgen synthesis and blocks the action of androgens at the receptor level. It is widely used to treat hirsutism in women. It is only moderately effective, and a decrease in hair growth may be noted only after 3 to 6 months of treatment.

- Estrogen–progesterone combination therapy is sometimes helpful, presumably through suppression of pituitary luteinizing hormone (LH) secretion, and also through stimulation of hepatic synthesis of sex-hormone binding globulin, which decreases the unbound fraction of testosterone.

- Glucocorticoids, given in physiologic doses that do not cause Cushing's syndrome, may decrease adrenal androgen production by suppressing ACTH. They also may decrease ovarian androgen production through an unknown mechanism.

Male Reproduction

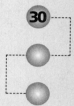

The Testes

The testes perform two main functions: they produce testosterone, which regulates male sexual development and function, and they produce spermatozoa. The hypothalamic–pituitary unit controls testosterone production through stimulation of the Leydig cells by luteinizing hormone (LH), and controls sperm production through the stimulation of the seminiferous tubule cells by follicle-stimulating hormone (FSH).

MORPHOLOGY OF THE TESTES

 The testicular parenchyma consists of coiled seminiferous tubules, surrounded by connective tissue that contains the Leydig cells (interstitial cells) as well as blood vessels and lymphatics (Fig. 30-1). The seminiferous tubules empty into a network of ducts, the rete testis, which drains into the epididymis; this in turn empties into the vas deferens, then the ejaculatory duct, and then the urethra.

- The seminiferous tubules are lined by Sertoli cells. Spermatogonia, the undifferntiated male germ cells, are interspersed with the Sertoli cells, and the process of spermatogenesis takes place between the Sertoli cells, in close proximity to their cytoplasm.

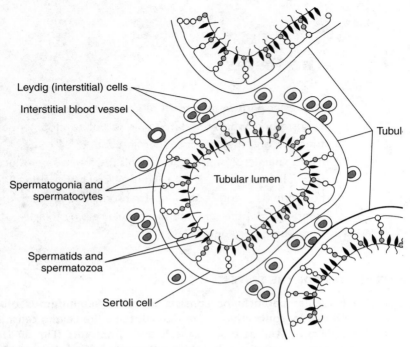

Leydig (interstitial) cells

Interstitial blood vessel

Tubul

Spermatogonia and
spermatocytes

Tubular lumen

Spermatids and
spermatozoa

Sertoli cell

Figure 30-1. Histologic section of a normal testis.

TESTICULAR HORMONES

 The Leydig cells in the interstitial tissues of the testis produce the testicular androgens. The synthetic pathways are similar to those in the adrenals and ovaries, but testosterone is the main product (Fig. 30-2).

■ LH stimulates androgen production by increasing the conversion of cholesterol to pregnenolone through side-chain cleavage. Testosterone may be converted to dihydrotestosterone in androgen target cells such as skin and prostate, and to estradiol in adipose tissue.

■ The actions of testosterone and other androgenic hormones are listed in Table 30-1. Testosterone (or in some tissues, dihydrotestosterone) produces these effects by binding to a specific androgen receptor located mainly in the nucleus of androgen-responsive cells. The hormone-receptor complex binds to DNA sequences, leading to

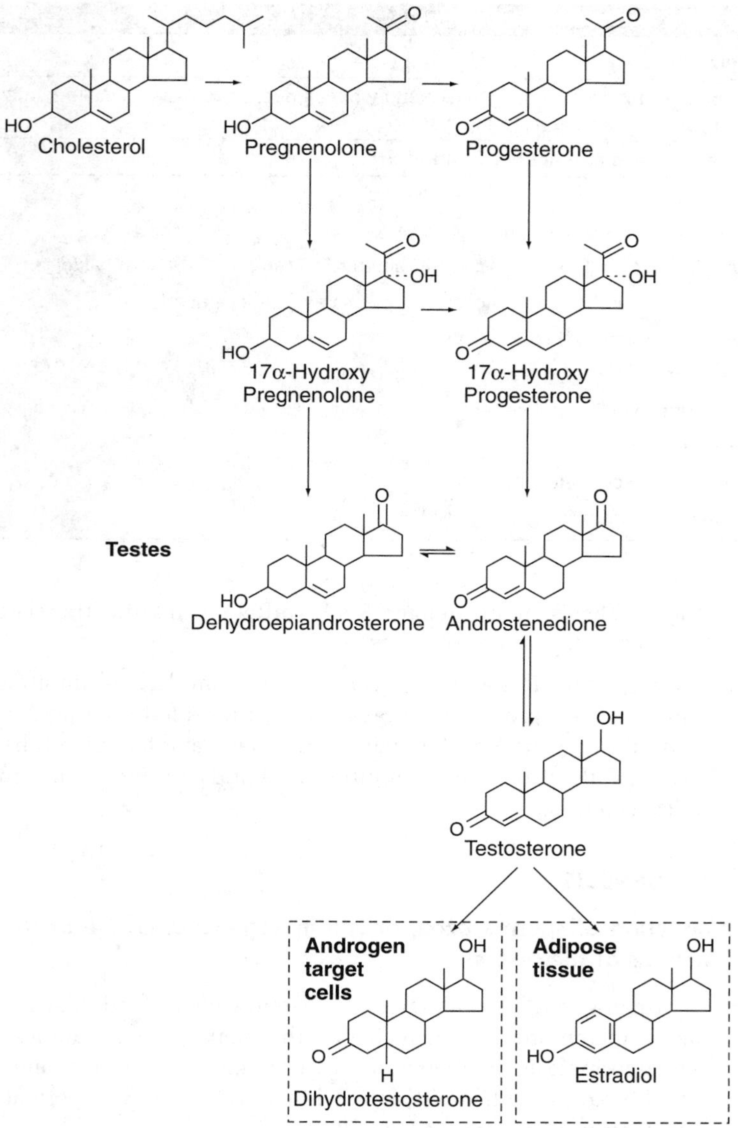

Figure 30-2. Biosynthesis of testicular hormones. Testosterone and androstenedione are the principal androgens produced by the testes. Testosterone is converted to dihydrotestosterone in some tissues by the enzyme 5α-reductase, and to estradiol in other tissues by the enzyme aromatase.

Table 30-1. Actions of Androgens

In utero

Development of male external genitalia and wolffian duct structures (epididymis, ductus deferens, seminal vesicles, ejaculatory duct)

Pubertal changes and actions in adult life

Growth of penis, testes, prostate, seminal vesicles

Enlargement of larynx, deepening of voice

Growth of pubic, axillary, and facial hair; potential to cause male-pattern baldness

Linear growth spurt at puberty, followed by closure of the epiphyses

Maintenance of bone mineral density

Increase in muscle mass, male body configuration

More aggressive behavioral pattern

Sexual potency

Maintenance of spermatogenesis

Stimulation of erythropoiesis

the synthesis of messenger RNA (mRNA) and the translation of androgen-dependent proteins.

- During fetal life the Sertoli cells produce müllerian-inhibiting hormone, a glycoprotein that causes regression of the müllerian ducts and thus prevents development of the uterus and fallopian tubes. The Sertoli cells also produce inhibin, a peptide hormone that inhibits FSH secretion.

SPERMATOGENESIS

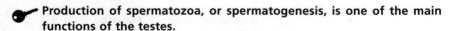 **Production of spermatozoa, or spermatogenesis, is one of the main functions of the testes.**

- Spermatogonia are undifferentiated stem cells located near the basement membrane of the cells of the seminiferous tubules. They undergo meiosis, or reduction of the number of chromosomes from the diploid to the haploid state, while developing into spermatocytes and then into spermatids (Fig. 30-3).
- Transformation of spermatids into spermatozoa involves nuclear and cytoplasmic changes and formation of the flagellum. As these cells

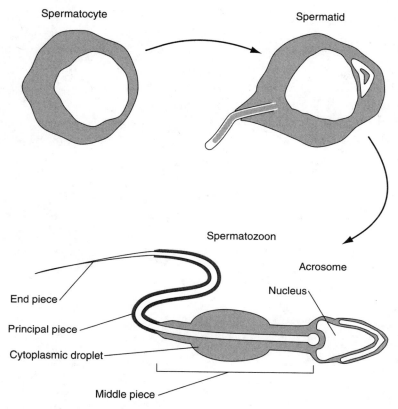

Figure 30-3. Stages in the formation of a spermatozoon.

differentiate, they move toward the lumen of the tubules, where the
spermatozoa are released.

■ Formation of spermatozoa from spermatogonia requires about
70 days, and transport to the ejaculatory duct requires an additional
14 days. Sperm formation is stimulated by the actions of FSH and
testosterone on the Sertoli cells, which affect the process of spermatogenesis through the close contact of their cytoplasm with the
developing sperm cells.

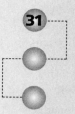

Male Hypogonadism

Inadequacy of testicular function (eunuchoidism) can affect sexual function, which depends on testosterone production, and fertility, which depends on sperm production. Testosterone levels may be returned to normal by parenteral or transdermal administration of this hormone, but restoration of fertility may or may not be possible.

CAUSES OF MALE HYPOGONADISM

🔑 Male hypogonadism is caused by disorders of the testes or of the hypothalamic–pituitary axis.

- In male hypogonadism caused by disorders of the hypothalamus or pituitary, a decrease in luteinizing hormone (LH) and follicle-stimulating hormone (FSH) production is the cause of the inadequate testicular function. This is called *hypogonadotropic hypogonadism* (Table 31-1).

Table 31-1. Causes of Hypogonadism in Men
Hypogonadotropic syndromes
Hypopituitarism (Panhypopituitarism or isolated gonadotropin deficiency)
Kallman's syndrome
Prolactin-producing pituitary adenoma
Delayed puberty
Hypergonadotropic syndromes
Klinefelter's syndrome
Testicular agenesis
Testicular injury
Mumps orchitis
Other infections (e.g., gonorrhea)
Trauma
Surgery
Radiotherapy, chemotherapy
Cryptorchidism

- In primary disorders of the testes, LH and FSH are elevated because the diminished circulating testosterone level leads to decreased negative-feedback effects on the hypothalamus and pituitary. This is referred to as *hypergonadotropic hypogonadism* (see Table 31-1).

- Kallman's syndrome is a form of hypogonadotropic hypogonadism caused by a congenital defect in the hypothalamus. It is associated with midline defects such as agenesis of the olfactory lobes, causing anosmia.

- Puberty may occur spontaneously up to about age 20. Until then, one may suspect delayed puberty, based on a family history of late sexual maturation, but a definite diagnosis of delayed puberty rather than permanent hypogonadism is made only after the occurrence of spontaneous puberty.

- Klinefelter's syndrome is a chromosomal disorder (typically 47,XXY) that results in a decrease in size of the testes, with hyalinization of the seminiferous tubules and azoospermia. Gynecomastia is common, and androgen deficiency may be caused by decreased Leydig cell function.

MANIFESTATIONS AND TREATMENT OF MALE HYPOGONADISM

Diagnosis of male hypogonadism is based on measurement of levels of testosterone, LH, and FSH. Imaging studies may be needed to rule out pituitary adenoma. Male hypogonadism is treated with testosterone.

- If testosterone deficiency prevents the occurrence of puberty, secondary sex characteristics do not develop.

  - The voice remains high-pitched, the penis and testes remain small, and other pubertal changes may not occur.

  - Without the effect of testosterone in causing closure of the epiphyses, the growth of long bones is relatively increased, causing the "eunuchoid habitus": the arm span is more than 2 inches greater than the height, and the heel-to-symphysis pubis distance is more than 2 inches greater than the symphysis-to-crown distance.

- If testosterone deficiency begins after puberty, men may present with a decrease in potency and libido.

  - Loss of muscle strength, decreased facial hair growth, and infertility may be present, but other secondary sex characteristics such as deepening of the voice do not regress once pubertal changes have occurred.

- Detection of a low serum testosterone level (especially free testosterone, the fraction not bound to sex-hormone binding globulin) confirms the diagnosis of hypogonadism.

  • Measurement of levels of LH and FSH determines whether the origin of the problem is in the hypothalamic–pituitary axis (low levels of FSH and LH) or in the testes (elevated levels of FSH and LH).

  • If hypogonadotropic hypogonadism is found, magnetic resonance imaging (MRI) of the pituitary, with contrast, should be done because pituitary adenomas are a common cause of this condition. Prolactin should be measured for the same reason.

- Male hypogonadism is treated with testosterone, which is effective in restoring secondary sexual characteristics.

  • Oral administration is not effective because testosterone is inactivated by its initial passage through the liver. Instead, the hormone is injected as a depot preparation at 2- to 4-week intervals. Alternatively, testosterone may be used daily in the form of a patch or gel applied to the skin; this method allows transdermal absorption.

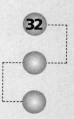

32 Gynecomastia

Enlargement of the male breast is caused by diverse disorders and medications, and by such common conditions as puberty, obesity, and old age. These causes have in common an increase in the ratio of estrogenic-to-androgenic effects on breast tissue, either because of increased estrogenic or decreased androgenic effect.

■ Pubertal gynecomastia occurs in two thirds of normal boys at 12 to 15 years of age, and disappears in most cases within 6 to 24 months. When gynecomastia persists, however, reduction mammoplasty must be considered if the breast enlargement causes severe psychologic stress.

■ Drugs that may cause gynecomastia include estrogens (used, for example, in the treatment of prostate cancer), spironolactone, cimetidine, digitalis, phenothiazines, tricyclic antidepressants, methyldopa, reserpine, isoniazid, and marijuana. Mechanisms include direct estrogenic effect, and inhibition of the binding of androgen to its receptor.

■ Obesity and aging, with increased body stores of adipose tissue, may be associated with gynecomastia. Increased androgen conversion to estrogen in adipose tissue is thought to be responsible (see Fig. 30-2).

■ Alcoholic cirrhosis and other liver diseases may cause gynecomastia because of increased peripheral androgen-to-estrogen conversion.

• Alcohol also may inhibit testosterone production and increase hepatic metabolism of testosterone.

■ Gynecomastia, usually self-limited, may be associated with refeeding after a period of starvation. This may reflect increased sensitivity of breast tissue to sex steroids after the prolonged hypogonadotropic hypogonadism that occurs with starvation.

• A similar mechanism may explain pubertal gynecomastia.

■ Gonadotropin excess may cause gynecomastia by stimulating aromatase in the Leydig cells, leading to increased estrogen production relative to testosterone. This occurs in primary hypogonadism, or with tumors of the liver or testis that produce human chorionic gonadotropin.

■ Other causes of gynecomastia include renal failure and estrogen-producing tumors of the adrenal or testis.

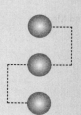

Study Questions

DIRECTIONS: Each of the numbered items or incomplete statements in this section is followed by answers or by completions of the statement. Select the ONE lettered answer or completion that is BEST in each case.

1. A patient suffers damage to the pituitary stalk during surgery to remove a tumor in the hypothalamic area. Which pituitary hormone might be expected to increase rather than decrease in serum concentration?
   (A) Adrenocorticotropic hormone (ACTH)
   (B) Thyroid-stimulating hormone (TSH)
   (C) Growth hormone (GH)
   (D) Prolactin
   (E) Luteinizing hormone (LH)

2. A 40-year-old woman notes increased frequency of urination. Her fasting serum glucose level is normal. Which of the following findings would suggest a diagnosis of primary polydipsia?
   (A) Urine specific gravity of 1.005 (low)
   (B) Urine osmolality of 190 mOsm/kg (low)
   (C) Serum osmolality of 264 mOsm/kg (low)
   (D) A history of recent head injury
   (E) A serum sodium concentration of 150 mmol/L (high)

Questions 3–7
   For each numbered item, select the one lettered option that is most closely associated with it.
   (A) Hypopituitarism
   (B) Pituitary tumor
   (C) Acromegaly
   (D) Galactorrhea–amenorrhea syndrome
   (E) Cushing's disease
   (F) Central diabetes insipidus
   (G) Syndrome of inappropriate antidiuretic hormone (ADH)

3. Hyponatremia

4. Rapid response to treatment with a dopamine agonist

5. Bitemporal hemianopsia

6. Enlargement of the mandible

7. Nonpitting edema

Questions 8–10

For each numbered item, select the one lettered option that is most closely associated with it.

   (A) Thyroxine (T_4)
   (B) Triiodothyronine (T_3)
   (C) Thyrotropin
   (D) Thyroglobulin
   (E) Thyroid peroxidase

8. The most active form of thyroid hormone

9. The main component of the colloid of the thyroid follicle

10. The main product of the thyroid gland

11. A healthy 27-year-old woman feels a lump in her neck. Examination shows this to be a 3-cm thyroid nodule. A fine-needle aspiration biopsy (FNA) of the nodule is performed. A radionuclide scan of the thyroid should be done if the FNA shows which of the following?
   (A) Sheets of follicular cells, suggesting a follicular neoplasm
   (B) Sample inadequate for interpretation
   (C) Normal follicular cells and colloid; no suspicion of malignancy
   (D) Abnormal cells indicative of thyroid cancer
   (E) Lymphocytic infiltration compatible with chronic autoimmune thyroiditis (Hashimoto's disease)

12. A diagnosis of subclinical hypothyroidism is made when a patient has which of the following?
   (A) Low thyroid hormone levels but no symptoms
   (B) Classic symptoms of hypothyroidism but normal thyroid function test results
   (C) Low free T_4 levels but normal serum thyroid-stimulating hormone (TSH) level
   (D) Low serum TSH but normal free T_4 levels
   (E) Increased serum TSH but normal free T_4 levels

13. A 52-year-old woman complains of fatigue, weight gain, and constipation. Which of the following laboratory findings would provide the most convincing evidence that she suffers from hypothyroidism?
    (A) Decreased serum T_4
    (B) Decreased serum free T_3
    (C) Decreased T_3-resin uptake
    (D) Increased serum thyroid-stimulating hormone (TSH)
    (E) High titer of antithyroid peroxidase antibody

14. A young woman complains of nervousness and difficulty sleeping. Her serum total T_4 level is elevated. Which of the following would be evidence against a diagnosis of hyperthyroidism?
    (A) A decrease in the serum level of thyroid-stimulating hormone (TSH)
    (B) An increase in the serum level of triiodothyronine (total T_3)
    (C) A decrease in T_3-resin uptake
    (D) An increased level of anti–TSH-receptor antibody
    (E) An increase in thyroidal radioiodine uptake

Questions 15–17
    For each numbered item, select the one lettered option that is most closely associated with it.
    (A) Graves' disease
    (B) Hypothyroidism
    (C) Subacute thyroiditis
    (D) Chronic autoimmune thyroiditis
    (E) Estrogen therapy

15. Very high concentration of antithyroid peroxidase antibody

16. Increased serum free T_4, decreased serum thyroid-stimulating hormone (TSH), decreased thyroidal radioiodine uptake

17. Increased total T_4, decreased T_3-resin uptake

18. A 35-year-old man complains of nausea and malaise, and is diagnosed with primary hyperparathyroidism. Surgical exploration of the neck is performed, and a small parathyroid adenoma is found and removed. Which of the following would provide the strongest evidence that the disease has been cured?
    (A) The surgeon found a normal-sized parathyroid gland on the same side as the adenoma.
    (B) The patient develops mild hypocalcemia 8 hours after the operation.
    (C) The patient's symptoms are relieved the day after surgery.

(D) The removed adenoma proves to be benign on histologic examination.

(E) Serum calcium levels were only slightly elevated before surgery.

Questions 19–21

For each numbered item, select the one lettered option that is most closely associated with it.

(A)   Primary hypoparathyroidism
(B)   Primary hyperparathyroidism
(C)   Pseudohypoparathyroidism
(D)   Osteoporosis
(E)   Osteomalacia
(F)   Hypercalcemia of malignancy

19. Positive Chvostek sign and elevated serum parathyroid hormone (PTH) level

20. Loss of bone matrix and bone mineral density, and normal serum calcium level

21. Elevated serum calcium level and elevated serum PTH level

22. A 60-year-old woman is found on routine examination to have a serum calcium of 11.1 mg/dL (mildly elevated). The serum parathyroid hormone (PTH) level is elevated, and primary hyperparathyroidism is diagnosed. The woman is asymptomatic. Which of the following would indicate that surgical treatment should be recommended?

(A) The serum calcium remains slightly elevated, ranging from 10.6 to 11.2 mg/dL.

(B) The serum PTH level remains high.

(C) Bone mineral density at the hip is 2.5 SD below the expected peak bone mass at age 30.

(D) Urine calcium excretion is 200 mg/24 hours (normal: up to 250 mg/ 24 hours).

(E) An early cataract is noted in the right eye.

23. The kidneys play the principal role in which step in the synthesis of the active form of vitamin D?

(A) Conversion of 7-dehydrocholesterol to vitamin D_3

(B) Absorption of vitamin D_2

(C) Conversion of vitamin D to 25-OH vitamin D

(D) Absorption of vitamin D_3

(E) Conversion of 25-OH vitamin D to 1,25-$(OH)_2$ vitamin D

24. Bone resorption is increased by which one of the following?
    (A) Estrogens
    (B) Calcitonin
    (C) Bisphosphonates
    (D) Hyperparathyroidism
    (E) Hypothyroidism

Questions 25–27
    For each numbered item, select the one lettered option that is most closely associated with it.
    (A) Increase β-cell secretion of insulin
    (B) Increase sensitivity of body tissues to insulin
    (C) Bind to insulin receptors and affect glucose metabolism
    (D) Slow the rate of intestinal absorption of glucose
    (E) Prolong the duration of action of insulin

25. α-Glucosidase inhibitors

26. Thiazolidinediones

27. Sulfonylureas

28. A 60-year-old man with type 2 diabetes mellitus develops progressive weakness and confusion over a 10-day period. In the emergency department, he is found to have dry skin and mucous membranes, and low blood pressure (100/60 mm Hg). Serum glucose is very high (950 mg/dL), but blood pH is normal (7.38), and his serum is negative for ketones. Serum osmolality is 335 mOsm/kg. The first priority in management is
    (A) intravenous insulin
    (B) intravenous pressor agents
    (C) fluid replacement
    (D) computed tomographic scan of the head
    (E) search for a precipitating cause

29. The earliest sign of diabetic nephropathy is
    (A) an increase in the serum blood urea nitrogen (BUN) level
    (B) an increase in the serum creatinine level
    (C) proteinuria
    (D) microalbuminuria
    (E) decreased urine output

30. Which one of the following contributes to the pathogenesis of diabetic ketoacidosis?
    (A) Increased peripheral utilization of glucose
    (B) Increased hepatic glucose output
    (C) Decreased release of amino acids from muscle
    (D) Decreased oxidation of triglycerides in fat cells
    (E) Decreased production of acetoacetate in the mitochondria of liver cells

31. A 27-year-old woman is diagnosed with diabetes mellitus. Which of the following findings would point most convincingly to type 1 rather than type 2 diabetes?
    (A) She is not obese.
    (B) Severe polydipsia and polyuria preceded the diagnosis.
    (C) Ketoacidosis was present at the time of diagnosis.
    (D) The serum C-peptide level was normal at the time of diagnosis.
    (E) Glucose levels rose above 600 mg/dL before treatment was started.

Questions 32–34
    For each numbered item, select the one lettered option that is most closely associated with it.
    (A) Type 1 diabetes mellitus
    (B) Type 2 diabetes mellitus
    (C) Impaired fasting glucose
    (D) Impaired glucose tolerance
    (E) Diabetic ketoacidosis
    (F) Hyperglycemic hyperosmolar nonketotic coma

32. Very high serum level of acetoacetate

33. Very high serum level of anti-islet cell antibodies

34. Plasma glucose level greater than 140 mg/dL, but less than 200 mg/dL, 2 hours after an oral load of 75 g of glucose

35. Type 1 diabetes mellitus is usually associated with which one of the following?
    (A) Onset in middle age
    (B) Obesity
    (C) Insulin resistance
    (D) Requirement for insulin therapy
    (E) Absence of autoimmune manifestations

36. The actions of insulin include which one of the following?
    (A) Increased utilization of glucose by muscle
    (B) Increased hepatic output of glucose
    (C) Increased lipolysis
    (D) Increased amino acid flux from muscle due to protein breakdown
    (E) Increased glycogenolysis

Questions 37–39
    For each numbered item, select the one lettered option that is most closely associated with it.
    (A) Fasting serum glucose level
    (B) Random serum glucose level
    (C) Serum glucose level 2 hours after a 75-g oral glucose load (oral glucose tolerance test)
    (D) Serum level of hemoglobin A_{1C}
    (E) Urine glucose concentration

37. The most sensitive test for diabetes mellitus

38. The recommended screening test for diabetes mellitus

39. The test that is most indicative of average recent blood glucose levels

40. In a normal person, which of the following would be associated with a decrease in the serum concentration of cortisol?
    (A) Blood sampling at 6 P.M. rather than 6 A.M.
    (B) An intravenous injection of insulin
    (C) Onset of an acute viral upper respiratory infection
    (D) An injury that causes acute loss of blood
    (E) An intravenous injection of corticotropin-releasing hormone (CRH)

Questions 41–43
    For each numbered item, select the one lettered option that is most closely associated with it.
    (A) Is produced by cells of neuroectodermal origin
    (B) Secretion stimulated by angiotensin II
    (C) Is produced in the inner zone (reticularis) of the adrenal cortex
    (D) Inhibits the inflammatory response
    (E) Causes sodium loss and potassium retention

41. Aldosterone

42. Epinephrine

43. Cortisol

44. A 50-year-old woman is diagnosed with Addison's disease (adrenal insuffi-
    ciency), and treatment with cortisol and fludrocortisone acetate (Florinef)
    is started. One month later she still complains of weakness and fatigue.
    Which of the following would suggest that the dose of Florinef should be
    increased?
    (A) Ankle edema
    (B) Increased blood pressure
    (C) Hyperkalemia
    (D) Hypernatremia
    (E) Increasing pigmentation

45. A young man is found to have hypertension. Pheochromocytoma is sus-
    pected because of paroxysmal episodes of symptoms, with blood pressure
    elevations up to 200/120 mm Hg during the paroxysms. Which of the fol-
    lowing findings would further support a diagnosis of pheochromocytoma?
    (A) Central obesity, with a dorsal fat pad
    (B) Hypoglycemia
    (C) Low serum potassium level
    (D) Postural hypotension
    (E) Marked fall in blood pressure with spironolactone treatment

46. A 55-year-old man complains of fatigue, weight loss, and joint pains. Lab-
    oratory studies reveal that his serum cortisol level is undetectable. Which
    of the following findings would suggest most strongly that he has primary
    adrenal insufficiency rather than secondary adrenal insufficiency due to
    hypopituitarism?
    (A) Serum sodium and potassium levels are normal.
    (B) Serum free thyroxine levels are low.
    (C) Blood pressure is low, and decreases further when the patient stands up.
    (D) The patient has noted severe weakness and dizziness during upper
        respiratory infections.
    (E) The patient has noted some darkening of the exposed areas of his
        skin.

47. A 53-year-old woman has symptoms and physical findings of Cushing's
    syndrome, and her 24-hour urine free cortisol excretion is consistently
    high. Serum cortisol levels are not suppressed by standard low-dose dexa-
    methasone testing, but are suppressed normally by high-dose dexametha-
    sone testing. This suggests which of the following diagnoses?
    (A) Normal adrenal function
    (B) Cushing's disease due to a pituitary corticotroph adenoma
    (C) Cushing's syndrome due to an adrenal adenoma

(D) Ectopic adrenocorticotropic hormone (ACTH) syndrome

(E) Cushing's syndrome due to exogenous glucocorticoid therapy

48. A young woman is found to have elevated blood pressure readings of about 180/110 mm Hg, and her serum potassium level is 3.0 mmol/L (low). A diagnosis of primary aldosteronism would be most strongly supported by which of the following?

(A) A 3-cm adenoma is found in the left adrenal gland by magnetic resonance imaging (MRI).

(B) Plasma aldosterone levels and plasma renin activity are elevated.

(C) Plasma aldosterone levels are elevated and plasma renin activity is low.

(D) Both adrenal cortices are found to be enlarged on MRI.

(E) Adrenal vein catheterization shows an increased aldosterone concentration in the blood draining both adrenal glands.

Questions 49–51

For each numbered item, select the appropriate lettered option(s). Each lettered option may be selected once, more than once, or not at all. Each item will state the number of options to select; choose exactly this number.

(A) Testosterone

(B) Dihydrotestosterone

(C) Estrogen

(D) Luteinizing hormone (LH)

(E) Follicle-stimulating hormone (FSH)

(F) Gonadotropin-releasing hormone (GnRH)

49. Stimulation of the Leydig cells (select 1 hormone)

50. Growth of the prostate (select 1 hormone)

51. Spermatogenesis (select 2 hormones)

52. In the normal menstrual cycle, key events occur in which of the following sequences?

(A) Corpus luteum formation, rising estrogen levels, luteinizing hormone (LH) surge, ovulation

(B) Rising estrogen levels, ovulation, LH surge, corpus luteum formation

(C) Rising estrogen levels, LH surge, ovulation, corpus luteum formation

(D) Ovulation, rising estrogen levels, LH surge, corpus luteum formation

(E) LH surge, ovulation, rising estrogen levels, corpus luteum formation

53. A 17-year-old boy has not experienced any pubertal changes. He is 74 inches tall, and has an increased arm span and small testes. Levels of serum testosterone, luteinizing hormone (LH), and follicle-stimulating hormone (FSH) are low. Which of the following findings is most likely to be present?
    (A) Bilateral varicocele
    (B) Increased upper body-to-lower body ratio
    (C) Impaired sense of smell
    (D) Mental retardation
    (E) XXY karyotype

54. A 17-year-old girl has never had a menstrual period. She is 58 inches tall and has no signs of pubertal development. Levels of serum luteinizing hormone (LH) and follicle-stimulating hormone (FSH) are elevated. The most likely diagnosis is
    (A) pituitary tumor
    (B) 45X gonadal dysgenesis (Turner's syndrome)
    (C) congenital adrenal hyperplasia
    (D) hypothalamic amenorrhea
    (E) uterine abnormality

55. In a patient with hypothalamic amenorrhea, normal ovulatory menstrual cycles would most likely be restored by
    (A) estrogen administration for 21 days each month
    (B) estrogen administration for 25 days each month with progesterone added on days 16 to 25
    (C) gonadotropin-releasing hormone (GnRH) given by intravenous pulse injection every 2 hours
    (D) GnRH given by constant intravenous infusion
    (E) testosterone given as a depot injection every 2 weeks

56. A 27-year-old woman complains of oligomenorrhea (three periods in the past year) and excess facial hair growth. The findings of obesity, increased serum luteinizing hormone (LH) level, increased serum estrogen level, and insulin resistance would suggest which of the following diagnoses?
    (A) Congenital adrenal hyperplasia
    (B) Polycystic ovary syndrome
    (C) Hypothalamic amenorrhea
    (D) Kallman's syndrome
    (E) Virilizing ovarian tumor

57. A young woman is studied for infertility because she has been unable to become pregnant after 2 years of trying. Which of the following findings would most strongly indicate that ovulation is occurring?

     (A) Body temperature remains constant throughout the menstrual cycle.
     (B) Serum progesterone levels rise in the luteal phase of the cycle.
     (C) Serum estrogen levels rise in the luteal phase of the cycle.
     (D) Menstrual periods occur regularly every 30 days.
     (E) Serum levels of follicle-stimulating hormone (FSH) and luteinizing hormone (LH) are normal.

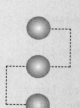

Answers and Explanations

1. **The correct answer is D.** Hypothalamic hormones reach the pituitary gland in high concentration after traveling down the pituitary stalk in the portal veins, and in general they stimulate pituitary hormone production. ACTH production is stimulated by corticotropin-releasing hormone (CRH), TSH production by thyrotropin-releasing hormone (TRH), and LH production by gonadotropin-releasing hormone (GnRH). Growth hormone is stimulated by growth hormone-releasing hormone (GHRH), whose effect predominates over the inhibitory effect of somatostatin. But the main effect of hypothalamic hormones on prolactin production is inhibitory, through the action of dopamine, and injury to the stalk that prevents dopamine from reaching the pituitary in high concentration may increase the secretion and blood concentration of prolactin.

2. **The correct answer is C.** In primary polydipsia the initial event is increased water intake, which lowers serum osmolality. In central diabetes insipidus, which is suggested by the history of head injury, the loss of free water in the urine causes an increase in serum osmolality and an increase in serum sodium concentration. Low urine osmolality and low urine specific gravity are present in both primary polydipsia (because of increased water intake) and central diabetes insipidus (because of antidiuretic hormone deficiency), so these changes do not help in differentiating between these two diagnoses.

3. **The correct answer is G.** The predominant clinical manifestation of the syndrome of inappropriate ADH is hyponatremia, which results both from the water retention and from the compensatory renal loss of sodium. The adrenal insufficiency associated with hypopituitarism, unlike primary adrenal insufficiency, is not usually associated with hyponatremia; aldosterone levels, controlled not by adrenocorticotropic hormone but by serum angiotensin II and potassium levels, are not reduced.

4. **The correct answer is D.** Whether the prolactin excess that causes the galactorrhea–amenorrhea syndrome is caused by medications, by a pituitary adenoma, or by another abnormality, it usually responds to drugs like bromocriptine and cabergoline that mimic the action of the natural hypothalamic prolactin-inhibiting factor, dopamine. Less often, pituitary

tumors other than prolactinomas may decrease in size and produce less hormone when dopamine agonists are given.

5. **The correct answer is B.** Pituitary macroadenomas (i.e., tumors larger than 10 mm in diameter) may grow upward and impinge on the central portion of the optic chiasm. This may impair the function of neuronal tracts to the medial half of each retina, causing bitemporal hemianopsia.

6. **The correct answer is C.** Excess production of growth hormone by a somatotroph adenoma causes characteristic skeletal changes, including enlargement of the mandible. Other skeletal effects are enlargement of the nose, the supraorbital ridges, and the hands and feet.

7. **The correct answer is A.** Nonpitting edema is characteristic of hypothyroidism, which may occur as a result of thyroid-stimulating hormone deficiency in hypopituitarism, as well as in primary thyroid disease. The firm tissue swelling does not easily pit with pressure because it is caused by mucopolysaccharide infiltration in the subcutaneous tissues rather than by the water accumulation that occurs in more common edematous states such as congestive heart failure or hepatic cirrhosis.

8. **The correct answer is B.** Triiodothyronine (T_3) binds to the intracellular receptors that in turn bind to nuclear DNA and bring about the actions of thyroid hormone. Thyroxine (T_4) can be considered a prohormone that must be converted to T_3 (in the liver or other extrathyroidal tissues) to exert its effect.

9. **The correct answer is D.** Thyroglobulin is a large protein, located mainly in the colloid of the thyroid follicle, that serves as a framework for the synthesis and then the storage of T_3 and T_4.

10. **The correct answer is A.** The thyroid gland secretes mainly thyroxine (T_4), much of which is converted to the active form of thyroid hormone, triiodothyronine (T_3), in peripheral tissues.

11. **The correct answer is A.** Because a follicular neoplasm may be an adenoma or a carcinoma, surgical removal may be necessary to make the distinction. Therefore, a radionuclide scan may be helpful, because finding the nodule to be hyperfunctioning on scan would justify a diagnosis of benign adenoma and avoid surgery. The decisions for nonsurgical management of a nodule with benign cytology or findings of Hashimoto's disease, or surgical removal of a nodule with malignant cytology, are unlikely to be altered by a radionuclide scan. If the FNA yields insufficient material, the procedure must be repeated.

12. **The correct answer is E.** The term "subclinical hypothyroidism" has come to refer specifically to an early stage in the development of hypothyroidism in which the serum TSH level has risen above normal, but the free T_4 level has not yet fallen below normal. The presence or absence of symptoms of hypothyroidism is not considered in the diagnosis, although it may influence the decision whether or not to treat with thyroid hormone.

13. **The correct answer is D.** Conditions other than hypothyroidism that raise serum TSH levels are very uncommon. The other choices are less specific indicators of hypothyroidism. Although the total T_4 level falls in hypothyroidism, it also may be decreased in persons with diminished thyroid hormone-binding proteins. Serum free T_3 levels may fall because of decreased T_4-to-T_3 conversion in persons with nonthyroidal illness or undernutrition. A decrease in the T_3-resin uptake may be caused by an increase in T_4-binding proteins. High levels of antithyroid peroxidase antibody indicate chronic autoimmune thyroiditis, but give no information on whether hypothyroidism is present.

14. **The correct answer is C.** A low T_3-resin uptake indicates an increase in unsaturated binding sites for thyroid hormone on the thyroid hormone-binding proteins; this suggests either an increase in these proteins or the presence of hypothyroidism, but not hyperthyroidism. Suppression of TSH (negative-feedback effect), increased serum total T_3, the presence of anti–TSH-receptor antibodies, and increased radioiodine uptake all are expected findings in Graves' disease.

15. **The correct answer is D.** Although low levels of antithyroid peroxidase antibodies, or antithyroglobulin antibodies, or both may be present in other autoimmune thyroid disesases, high titers strongly suggest chronic autoimmune thyroiditis (Hashimoto's disease).

16. **The correct answer is C.** The increased free T_4 and decreased TSH indicate thyrotoxicosis, which could be caused by Graves' disease or by subacute thyroiditis. But the decreased radioiodine uptake, indicating a decrease in function of the thyroid follicular cells, points to the diagnosis of subacute thyroiditis; in this condition, the cells are injured and thyroid hormone is passively released into the circulation.

17. **The correct answer is E.** A change in opposite directions of the total T_4 and T_3-resin uptake suggests an abnormality in thyroid hormone-binding proteins. Increased estrogen levels increase hepatic production of thyroxine-binding globulin, which raises the total T_4 and lowers the T_3-resin uptake.

18. **The correct answer is B.** Transient hypocalcemia after surgery strongly suggests that the remaining parathyroid glands have been suppressed by prolonged hypercalcemia. This would be expected if the remaining parathyroid glands are normal, but not if the underlying disease is parathyroid hyperplasia involving more than one gland. The latter possibility is not ruled out by finding one normal gland, because one or both of the glands on the contralateral side may be abnormal. Similarly, relief of symptoms (which may be transient), the preoperative calcium level, or the histologic appearance of the abnormal gland do not reliably distinguish adenoma from hyperplasia.

19. **The correct answer is C.** A positive Chvostek sign usually indicates hypocalcemia, which is present in both primary hypoparathyroidism and pseudohypoparathyroidism. But of these choices only pseudohypoparathyroidism, caused by end-organ insensitivity to PTH, is associated with normal or high, rather than low, PTH concentrations in blood.

20. **The correct answer is D.** Osteoporosis may be present in patients with primary hyperparathyroidism, but would be associated with hypercalcemia. The loss of bone matrix distinguishes this choice form osteomalacia, in which bone matrix is preserved but the mineral phase of bone is lost.

21. **The correct answer is B.** In hypercalcemia of malignancy the PTH level is not elevated, because the hypercalcemia is caused most often by PTH-related peptide. The other choices are not associated with hypercalcemia.

22. **The correct answer is C.** Bone mineral density that is 2.5 SD below the expected peak value at age 30 indicates osteoporosis. Bone density often increases after removal of a parathyroid adenoma, and low bone density is considered an indication for surgery. Mild elevations of serum calcium (up to 11.4 to 12.0 mg/dL) and increased serum PTH levels do not predict progressive disease, although progression may occur in a minority of patients. Hypercalciuria is a risk factor for renal stone disease, but normocalciuria does not favor a decision for surgery. Cataracts are associated with hypoparathyroidism, not hyperparathyroidism.

23. **The correct answer is E.** Absorption of vitamin D_2 and vitamin D_3 takes place in the small bowel, and conversion of 7-dehydrocholesterol to vitamin D_3 takes place in the skin. The liver converts vitamin D to 25-OH vitamin D, which is then converted to $1,25\text{-}(OH)_2$ vitamin D, the active form, by the kidneys.

24. **The correct answer is D.** Parathyroid hormone (PTH), in the persistently increased concentrations that are present in both primary and secondary

hyperparathyroidism, increases the action of osteoclasts in resorbing bone. Estrogens, calcitonin, and bisphosphonates all have the opposite effect and decrease bone resorption. Thyroid hormone excess, but not the deficiency seen in hypothyroidism, may act like PTH and increase bone resorption.

25. **The correct answer is D.** By inhibiting the splitting of oligosaccharides by α-glucosidase in the intestinal mucosa, these drugs slow the absorption of carbohydrates. This blunts the postprandial rise in blood glucose.

26. **The correct answer is B.** Thiazolidinediones bind to the peroxisome proliferator-activated receptor (PPAR), increasing the expression of glucose transporters and stimulating the action of insulin.

27. **The correct answer is A.** Sulfonylureas bind to receptors in the β-cells in the islets of Langerhans and cause an increase in the secretion of insulin by these cells.

28. **The correct answer is C.** This patient has hyperglycemic hyperosmolar nonketotic coma. Fluid replacement to correct hypovolemia should protect against the threats of shock and thromboembolism, raise the blood pressure, and lessen the hyperglycemia and hyperosmolality by improving renal function. Insulin should be given after fluid replacement has been started to further correct the hyperglycemia.

29. **The correct answer is D.** Urinary excretion of 30 to 300 mg of albumin in 24 hours is the earliest clinical warning of diabetic nephropathy. Progression to proteinuria (more than 300 mg of protein in 24 hours) and renal failure may follow.

30. **The correct answer is B.** Decreased insulin action leads to greater hepatic output of glucose, contributing to the hyperglycemia. Insulin deficiency also causes decreased (not increased) peripheral glucose utilization, and increased (not decreased) protein catabolism, lipolysis, and hepatic ketogenesis.

31. **The correct answer is C.** Diabetic ketoacidosis occurs only in type 1 diabetes. Normal or low body weight is much more common in type 1 diabetes, but does not rule out type 2 disease. Polyuria, polydipsia, and severe elevations in blood glucose levels may be seen in both type 1 and type 2 diabetes. The absence of C-peptide, not its presence, points to type 1 disease.

32. **The correct answer is E.** Acetoacetate, β-hydroxybutyrate, and acetone are the ketones that accumulate in type 1 diabetes, in the absence of adequate treatment, and produce the acute complication of diabetic ketoacidosis.

33. **The correct answer is A.** Type 1 diabetes mellitus is associated with evidence of autoimmune reactions directed against the β-cells of the islets of Langerhans. Anti-islet cell antibodies, anti-glutamic acid decarboxylase (anti-GAD), and other antibodies may be detected before and for a time after the onset of type 1 diabetes.

34. **The correct answer is D.** Impaired glucose tolerance is diagnosed when the glucose tolerance test results in a 2-hour glucose level higher than normal, but not high enough to indicate a diagnosis of diabetes mellitus.

35. **The correct answer is D.** Type 1 diabetes is characterized by an absolute, not relative, insulin deficiency, and insulin treatment is necessary. Onset later in life, obesity, and insulin resistance are more characteristic of type 2 diabetes. Anti-islet cell antibodies and other autoimmune manifestations are common at the onset of type 1 diabetes.

36. **The correct answer is A.** Insulin increases glucose utilization by muscle and other tissues, by promoting glucose entry into the cells and by other actions. Insulin promotes energy storage in the liver by increasing glycogen formation (not glycogenolysis or increased hepatic glucose output); in the fat cells by increasing fat storage (not lipolysis); and in muscle by increasing protein formation (not breakdown).

37. **The correct answer is C.** The ability to rapidly reduce serum glucose levels after a glucose load is lost earlier than the ability to lower glucose to normal over 8 to 12 hours. The oral glucose tolerance test therefore will identify more patients with early diabetes than a fasting glucose level.

38. **The correct answer is A.** Although a bit less sensitive than the oral glucose tolerance test, a fasting serum glucose level is much more easily obtained and therefore more effective as a screening test. A random serum glucose level is even more easily obtained, but has greater variability and therefore less specificity in the diagnosis of diabetes.

39. **The correct answer is D.** Hemoglobin A_{1C} levels depend on the average serum glucose levels over the previous 6 to 12 weeks, and therefore give information on average glycemic control that is not provided by a single fasting or post-glucose load determination. Urine glucose levels are influenced by the widely variable renal threshold for glucose and have little role in the diagnosis of diabetes.

40. **The correct answer is A.** Inborn diurnal variation in the activity of the hypothalamic–pituitary–adrenal axis leads to maximal cortisol production in the early morning, followed by a gradual decline in production until

about midnight. Insulin-induced hypoglycemia, infection, and injury are perceived as stress by higher cortical centers in the brain that then stimulate the hypothalamic–pituitary–adrenal axis, and cortisol levels are increased, not decreased. CRH also causes an increase, not decrease, in cortisol because it stimulates pituitary adrenocorticotropic hormone (ACTH) production, which in turn stimulates production of cortisol by the zona fasciculata of the adrenal cortex.

41. **The correct answer is B.** Aldosterone production in the outer zone (glomerulosa) of the adrenal cortex is controlled mainly by the renin–angiotensin system, not by adrenocorticotropic hormone (ACTH). Mineralocorticoids cause sodium retention (not loss) and potassium loss (not retention).

42. **The correct answer is A.** The adrenal medulla, which produces the adrenal catecholamines, differs from the adrenal cortex in its neuroectodermal rather than mesodermal origin.

43. **The correct answer is D.** Glucocorticoids are commonly used as pharmacologic agents because of their anti-inflammatory actions.

44. **The correct answer is C.** Florinef is a mineralocorticoid, which causes potassium excretion and sodium retention, so hyperkalemia suggests that more Florinef is needed. Edema, increased blood pressure, and hypernatremia suggest the opposite, that is, sodium retention related to an excessive dose of the mineralocorticoid. Increasing pigmentation suggests inadequate replacement of glucocorticoid, not mineralocorticoid.

45. **The correct answer is D.** Hypotension with standing, despite supine hypertension, may be seen in some patients with pheochromocytoma. This may be related to down-regulation of the adrenergic receptors necessary to maintain blood pressure with standing. Central obesity is characteristic of Cushing's syndrome; weight loss would be more common in a patient with a pheochromocytoma. Serum glucose tends to be raised, not lowered, by catecholamines. Hypokalemia, and response to spironolactone, are seen with primary aldosteronism, not pheochromocytoma.

46. **The correct answer is E.** Increased pigmentation occurs in patients with primary adrenal insufficiency because melanocyte-stimulating hormone (MSH) is increased when secretion of adrenocorticotropic hormone (ACTH) is stimulated by the negative-feedback effect of low serum cortisol concentrations. This cannot occur if failure of the pituitary corticotroph cells is the cause of the adrenal insufficiency. Normal mineralocorticoid action (as evidenced by normal serum sodium and potassium

levels) and the presence of inadequate function of other pituitary target organs (such as hypothyroidism) are suggestive of secondary, not primary, adrenal insufficiency. Postural hypotension and inability to tolerate stressful illness are seen in both primary and secondary adrenal insufficiency.

47. **The correct answer is B.** The ability to suppress ACTH production (and hence serum cortisol levels) in response to high-dose dexamethasone but not low-dose dexamethasone is characteristic of pituitary corticotroph adenomas. A normal hypothalamic–pituitary–adrenal axis is suppressed even by low doses of dexamethasone. In Cushing's syndrome caused by an adrenal adenoma, by the ectopic ACTH syndrome, or by exogenous glucocorticoids, cortisol levels are not significantly affected by either low or high doses of dexamethasone.

48. **The correct answer is C.** Only if the increased aldosterone production is a primary event, as is the case when the cause is an adrenal adenoma, will the resulting volume expansion lead to suppression of plasma renin activity. A finding of elevated plasma renin activity would suggest that the aldosterone elevation is secondary to something that stimulates renin production, such as volume contraction. Adrenal adenomas may produce hormones other than aldosterone, or may be inactive. Bilateral adrenal hyperplasia and bilateral excessive adrenal production of aldosterone may be associated with secondary as well as primary aldosteronism.

49. **The correct answer is D.** LH stimulates the Leydig cells (the interstitial cells of the testes) to synthesize testosterone.

50. **The correct answer is B.** Testosterone acts as a prohormone in the prostate. It is converted to dihydrotestosterone by the enzyme 5α-reductase, and it is the dihydrotestosterone that binds to nuclear receptors and stimulates growth of the prostate. Dihydrotestosterone is also the primary androgen that acts on the skin and some other tissues.

51. **The correct answers are A and E.** The Sertoli cells of the seminiferous tubules of the testes are stimulated by both FSH and testosterone, leading to maturation of the spermatogonia into spermatozoa.

52. **The correct answer is C.** As the dominant follicle grows in the follicular phase of the cycle, it produces increasing amounts of estrogen, which triggers a surge in LH. This surge causes ovulation, with release of the ovum and transformation of the remaining follicle into the corpus luteum.

53. **The correct answer is C.** This patient has hypogonadotropic hypogonadism, which in one form (Kallman's syndrome) is associated with

anosmia. Mental retardation and XXY karyotype may be associated with Klinefelter's sydrome, which is a form of *hyper*gonadotropic hypogonadism, not *hypo*gonadotropic hypogonadism. Bilateral varicocele may cause testicular damage, which also would cause *hyper*gonadotropic hypogonadism. Lack of sex steroids delays closure of the epiphyses of the long bones, which leads to a *decreased,* not *increased,* upper body-to-lower body ratio, because the long bones of the legs are affected more than the vertebrae and skull.

54. **The correct answer is B.** In Turner's syndrome, serum LH and FSH are elevated because of the negative-feedback effect of low estrogen levels. If primary amenorrhea is caused by pituitary or hypothalamic disease, the LH and FSH levels are low or normal. Anatomic abnormalities of the genital tract, or adrenal overproduction of androgens, also might cause primary amenorrhea but would not be associated with increased levels of gonadotropins.

55. **The correct answer is C.** Pulse injection of GnRH at 90- to 120-minute intervals leads to a normal physiologic pattern of pituitary secretion of luteinizing hormone (LH) and follicle-stimulating hormone (FSH), and may be followed by regular ovulatory menstrual cycles. Constant GnRH administration causes inhibition rather than stimulation of LH and FSH secretion. Estrogen administration, alone or with cyclic progesterone, may result in withdrawal bleeding but not in ovulation. Testosterone administration might inhibit, not stimulate, follicle development and ovulation.

56. **The correct answer is B.** Obesity, insulin resistance, increased serum LH (and normal or low FSH) levels, and increased serum estrogen (as well as testosterone) levels are associated with the polycystic ovary syndrome. None of the other choices is closely associated with insulin resistance or obesity. Hypothalamic amenorrhea and Kallman's syndrome are not usually associated with androgen excess. Congenital adrenal hyperplasia and virilizing ovarian tumors cause androgen excess, but increased LH levels would not be expected.

57. **The correct answer is B.** An increase in serum progesterone during the second half of the cycle indicates that ovulation has occurred and a corpus luteum has formed, which is producing progesterone. Lack of an increase in basal body temperature would suggest that ovulation has not occurred. The levels of estrogen and the gonadotropins, and the regularity of the cycles, are not reliable indicators of whether or not ovulation has occurred.

Index